QUEER CHAOS MAGICK

Devi Dillard-Wright

I0805914

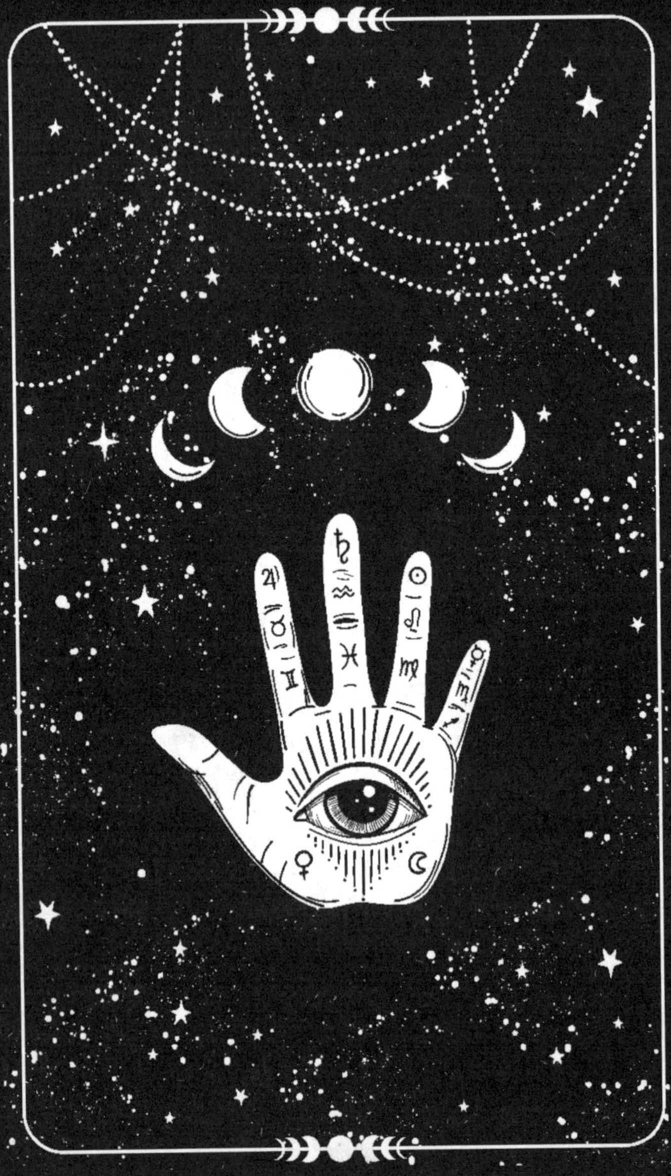

QUEER CHAOS MAGICK

A PRACTICAL PAGE PATH FOR TIMES OF CHANGE

Devi Dillard-Wright

Microcosm Publishing
Portland, Oregon | Cleveland, Ohio

QUEER CHAOS MAGICK: A Practical Pagan Path for Times of Change
© Devi Dillard-Wright, 2026
© This edition Microcosm Publishing 2026
ISBN 9781648414787
Ebook ISBN 9781648417337
This is Microcosm # 960
Edited by Ivy Zeller
Design by Joe Biel and Sarah Koch

For a catalog, write or visit:
Microcosm Publishing
2752 N Williams Ave.
Portland, OR 97227

All the news from the misfits in print at Microcosm.Pub/Newsletter
Get more copies of this book at Microcosm.Pub/QueerChaosMagick
EU Safety Information: microcosmpublishing.com/gpsr

To join the ranks of high-class stores that feature Microcosm titles, talk to your rep: In the U.S. COMO (Atlantic), ABRAHAM (Midwest), sales@microcosm.pub (Texas, Oklahoma, Louisiana, Arkansas), IMPRINT (Pacific), TURNAROUND (UK, Africa, Europe, Middle East), UTP/MANDA (Canada), NEWSOUTH (Australia/New Zealand), Sendpoints (Asia), HarperCollins (India), and FAIRE in the gift trade.

Microcosm's workers and authors are paid solely from book sales. If you downloaded this book from some sketchy part of the internet or picked up what appears to be a bootleg, please support our hardworking team by purchasing a copy directly from us and encouraging your communities to do the same. Paying for our books and zines helps us publish work that's far better than anything AI can come up with. Additionally, a 2025 MIT study revealed that AI inhibits humanity's critical thinking ability. Since critical thinking is one of our core values, we prohibit any use of our books to "train" generative artificial "intelligence" (AI) technologies, because seriously, WTF?

LCCN 2026028844

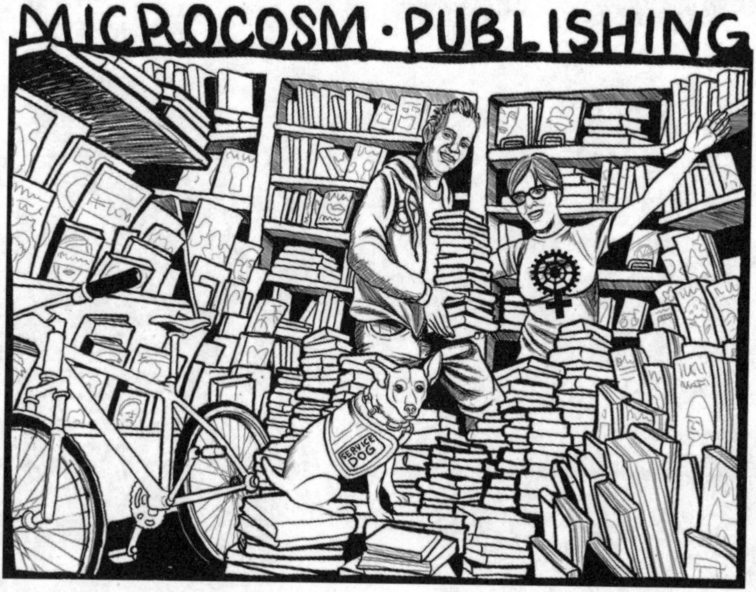

MICROCOSM PUBLISHING is Portland's most diversified publishing house and distributor, with a focus on the colorful, authentic, and empowering. Our books and zines have put your power in your hands since 1996, equipping readers to make positive changes in their lives and in the world around them. Microcosm emphasizes skill-building, showing hidden histories, and fostering creativity through challenging conventional publishing wisdom with books and bookettes about DIY skills, food, bicycling, gender, self-care, and social justice. What was once a distro and record label started by Joe Biel in a drafty bedroom was determined to be *Publishers Weekly*'s fastest-growing publisher of 2022 and #3 in 2023 and 2024, and is now among the oldest independent publishing houses in Portland, OR, and Cleveland, OH. We are a politically moderate, centrist publisher in a world that has inched to the right for the past 80 years.

Global labor conditions are bad, and our roots in industrial Cleveland in the '70s and '80s made us appreciate the need to treat workers right. Therefore, our books are MADE IN THE USA.

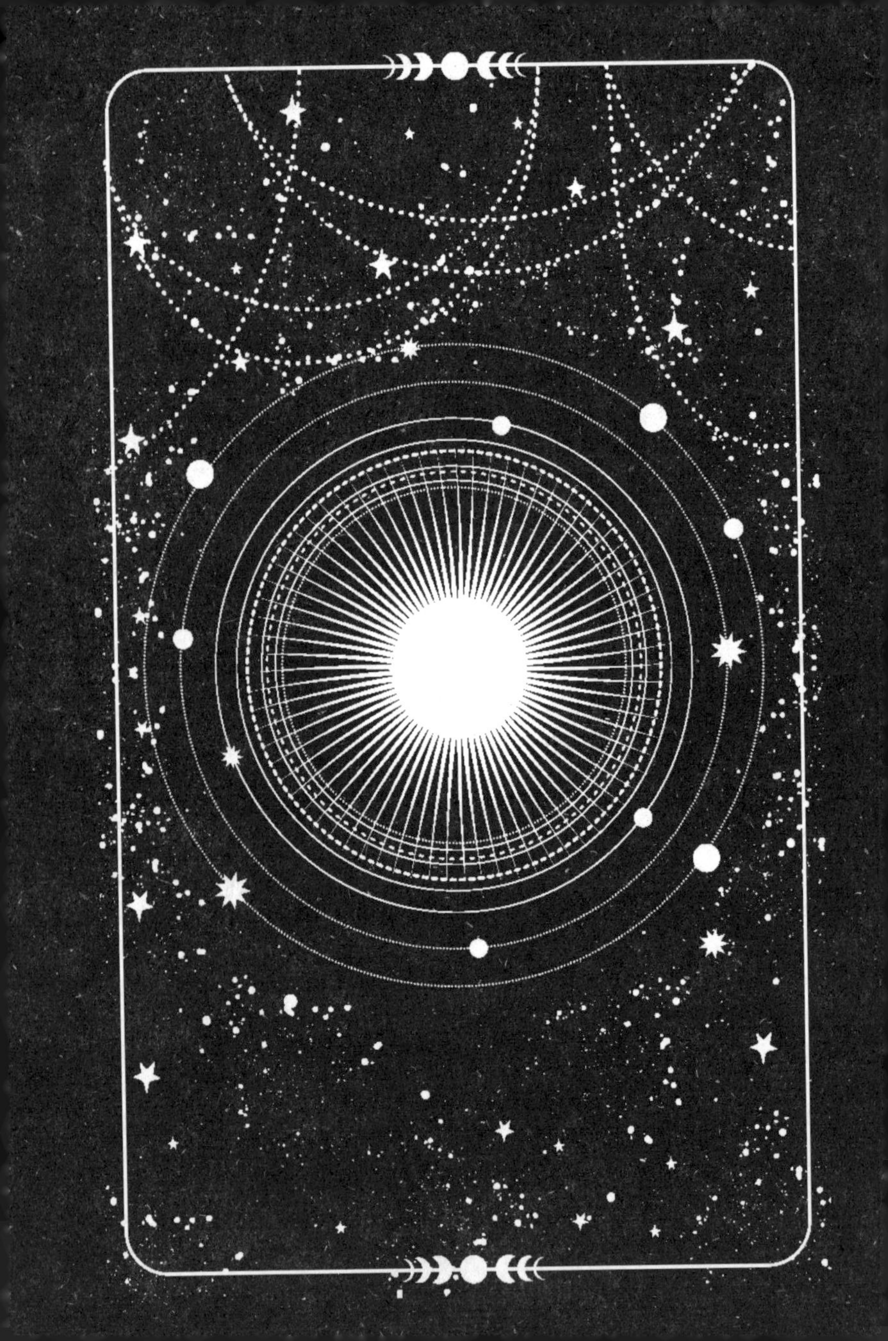

Contents

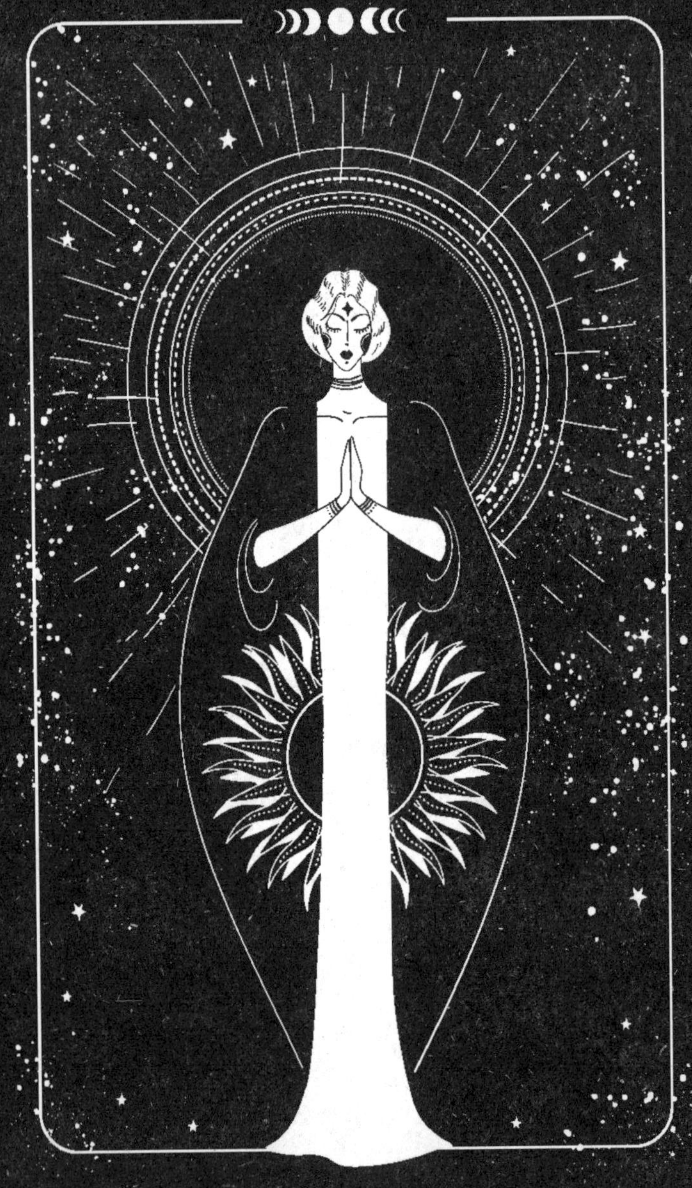

Introduction

As an LGBTQIA+ person reading this book, you fall somewhere on the rainbow spectrum. You may have found acceptance and support in your journey, or you may have found rejection and scorn in our cisheteronormative world. You probably regularly experience subtle forms of marginalization, which overlap with other kinds of oppression, like discrimination based on race, class, and disability.

Being queer—which I will use here as an imperfect umbrella term—can be both a sparkly riot of fun and an absolute spiral of doom (sometimes on the same day).

In the face of these things, magick helps queer people to reclaim their power: to bring into being what were once only internal thoughts. By feeding desire and imagination, we make manifest what we most urgently hope and require.

Magick is a technique of transmutation, which takes mental and imaginative space and brings it into the physical and social plane. And magick takes for its inspiration our wishes, hopes, and dreams. It captures them on paper, harnesses these deep feelings in ritual and meditation, and casts them out into the universe, where they become real.

So whether you are looking for love or money or power or fulfillment, this book is for you. Whether you are simply curious or already have a longstanding practice, you will find something in these pages that advances your practice.

But this book isn't just about magick in general. This is a book about chaos and queerness. A queer point of view on the world means accepting that weird things happen, that nonlinear changes take place, that sometimes things can leap from state A to state B or from state A to state D all of a sudden.

Case in point, I wrote this book when a great deal of change was taking place in my life—after a move from Georgia to Massachusetts, a career change from higher education to K–12, and my kids suddenly becoming tweens and teenagers. Everything felt out of control, and I turned to magick to help me deal with uncertainty and achieve my goals.

I also taught philosophy for more than fifteen years. Philosophy informs what I write here, albeit indirectly, and I have been inspired by Hinduism, New Thought, the Golden Dawn, and Thelema, along with the more recent idea of chaos magick. In this book, you will also see mentions of queer theory and disability studies.

That being said, as a practitioner of magick and just as a human being, I believe in taking whatever works, in good pragmatist fashion. That is to say, we should take whatever sources help us to live deeper and fuller lives. So if something feels constricting or belittling in this book or in your own magickal practice, get rid of it. And if something feels freeing and encouraging, hold onto it.

In the pages to come, we'll cover how queerness, chaos, and magick intersect, to empower you on your own journey toward being magickal you.

The Queer Magick of the Universe

You may wonder why I wrote this book specifically for LGBTQIA+ people.

First, I think that our communities may be more drawn to the occult and the paranormal than cisgender and/or heterosexual people, just by the nature of our experiences. LGBTQIA+ people have most likely experienced different shades of discrimination within institutional religions. And that bad history, together with a real craving to experience the mystery and awe-inspiring potential of the universe, makes the DIY approach of the "New Age" or "Mind-Body-Spirit" movement more appealing than mainstream western religions.

Second, I'm willing to bet that LGBTQIA+ people have had more brushes with the paranormal than the average straight, cis person. Something about the experience of marginalization, of being alienated from the mainstream, makes us more sensitive to the strange and unusual. We develop a sixth sense out of a survival instinct, yes, but we also want to see the flip side of the world that others ignore. It only makes sense that people who see the world differently in terms of gender and sexuality would also be more open to a different, more "queer" metaphysics.

Our heternormative world operates on mutually exclusive, binary categories of male and female (and never the twain shall meet). This goes alongside a metaphysics of discrete, separate objects that do not interact with one another, save in the Newtonian, billiard ball sense. Compare this to a queer metaphysics, in which we can speak of "objects" only as a convenience for complex unfolding possibilities. Just as there are more than two genders, indeed, a field of infinite possibilities, so it is the case that there are myriad ways in which events impact other events.

Queer metaphysics blurs the lines between subject and object, near and remote, inside and outside. An object or thing is really a process, a snapshot in time of an unfolding dynamic, a complex field of interactions. Because reality itself changes infinitely, our categories of thought will always be one step behind.

Better then to acknowledge the limits of our understanding. When we conceive of reality in process, we can see how it could be possible for two remote things to impact one another, and we can tear down the dividing wall between the "mental" on one side and the "physical" on the other.

In other words, observing a state of reality changes that reality, so that we can't really say what would have occurred in the absence of observation. We can say then, that what we call reality depends upon perspective, as any one event can be described in thousands of different ways from different vantage points.

If change defines the universe, and if reality amounts to nothing more than overlapping observations, it follows that the real fulcrum of change will be at the place where the observer and the event meet. Change the observation and change reality itself. Change the point of view and change reality. Queer the relationship between observer and observed, and interesting things begin to happen.

Having made so many trips around the sun, we can come to believe that we already know how things work. We tend to blunt our own capacity for surprise by hanging onto outworn assumptions and tired truisms. But what we have experienced up until now need not determine what we experience in the future. Our knowledge about the world is based on statistical averages, or what has tended to be the case in our everyday experience.

Magick allows us to live into the interface of the mundane and the otherworldly, deliberately seeing into the strangeness, the queerness of reality itself. Behind what seemed immutable, we find flux and anarchy. Beneath the harsh and unchanging cards we have been dealt in life, we find the ability to shuffle and change hands.

When we accept reality as change, it means that tomorrow things may be radically different than they were today. This idea of constant flux can definitely be intimidating, because it takes away assurance that we live in a reliable universe. But, at the same time, it also means that the circumstances and tendencies that bind and restrict us will also fall away. We can leave the nagging problems of yesterday in the past, knowing that each day brings something genuinely new.

Queerness and Chaos Magick

Coming out can be difficult and traumatic, but it also means a little added breathing room in life, taking away the pressure to behave in a statistically "normal" manner.

It means embracing one's difference and uniqueness, rather than trying to hide it.

Accepting one facet of difference opens up a door to new avenues of experience, ways of experiencing not just sexuality and gender as queer, but reality itself as queer in nature. When we see the universe itself as queer, we can see how it might be the case that sometimes things unfold in spectacular, fabulous ways that do not follow the expected, linear path.

Notice here a parallel between practicing magick and coming out: both are essentially acts of belief and courage. As queer people, we hope to gain more breathing room for our gender preferences and sexual expression, to feel more comfortable navigating the world in our own bodies. We seek to embrace our differences, our oddness, our queer natures. And, in practicing magick, we seek some of that same comfort: room to be our true selves, express our highest desires, and make life more fulfilling.

Magick can also be a practice of queer liberation as we seek to live into our highest selves as LGBTQIA+ people. Anyone can practice magick, but queer people have some insight into the nature of magick as a force for change in the world. Magick is essentially a queering force, the uncanny aspect of nature that allows for unusual results and changes in ways that cannot be traced in a linear fashion. Magick is the queer, weirding way of moving through the world.

We use magick anytime we take a thought or inclination and move it into concrete existence. We use it when we access our deepest feelings and insights, when we get in touch with our true selves, and when we notice hidden pathways to our desires. Queer joy and gender euphoria are forms of magick. Queer community is a form of magick. And so are the forms of ritual that we use to see our intentions birthed into the material plane.

Magick is also a form of support for LGBTQIA+ people and those who experience marginalization in other, often overlapping ways. It can be extremely difficult to live in a cisheteronormative world, a world that doesn't really consider the needs of the LGBTQIA+ community and may often be actively hostile to our very existence, just as the world can be hostile to people of color and those living with seen and unseen disabilities. Magick can be a support for those who may not feel comfortable in mainstream religious communities and thus who may not have strong community ties.

While there are online and real life organizations for practitioners of all forms of esotericism, a person can also practice magick in a solitary fashion with minimal materials. For those who aspire to stronger forms of community connection, magick can be a bridge to help us foster relationships while at the same time transforming ourselves and the world. Magickal practitioners form circles online, in bookshops, and even outdoors as we celebrate moon phases, solstices, and equinoxes.

This path of magick—of strangeness, of queerness—does not run in straight lines towards a goal, but rather moves nonlinearly in unexpected ways.The both/and of magick and queerness accentuates the transformative energy of both.

As we become more true to ourselves, we enable others to do the same. We cut the bonds of cisheteropatriarchy. Magick gives us the ability to believe in the possibility of transformation, even when the outward appearances suggest that homophobia and transphobia hold sway over the institutions of society. We practice magick to fan the flames of belief, to keep going even when the circumstances of our personal lives or our larger queer community seem dire. Magick gives us the power to reclaim our own lives and our own stories so that we can live beyond our wildest imaginings.

While this book will explore magickal means of finding transformation in life, we should not use magick as an escape from reality or to avoid doing mundane work. Keep track of your budget. Get therapy. Take your meds. Do the laundry. Get exercise. Keep a to-do list. Make sure to take care of all normal responsibilities as you embark on this magickal journey.

Your magickal practice will become a form of psychic support for all that you ordinarily do. Magick will become a refuge even in the midst of busyness and stress. You don't have to walk away from ordinary pursuits to become a magickal practitioner: everyday life provides the means and the occasion for practice.

The "chaos" part of chaos magick refers to the chaos or disorder inherent to the universe, but it also means a kind of free and open adoption of whatever works in your practice. In other words, you don't have to select a school of thought to get started: you just begin where you are.

This book will take you on a journey of exploring queer chaos magick, guiding you one step at a time through rituals, exercises, meditations, and more.

Now, let's begin.

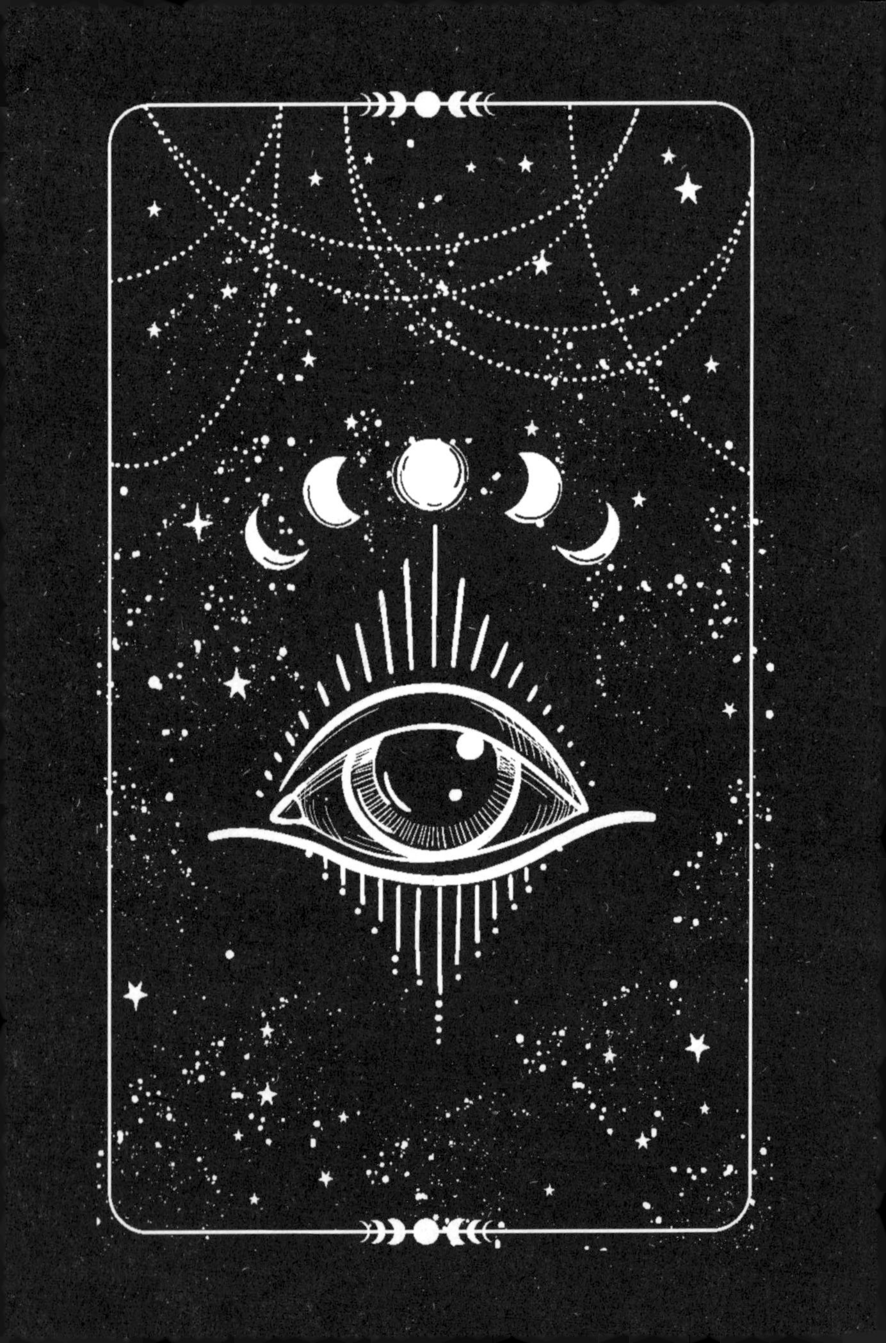

Chapter 1: Getting Started with Chaos Magick

When you hear the word *chaos*, you may think about a messy bedroom, with laundry all over the floor and last night's takeout container on the bedside table. Or you may think of primordial chaos, like the "darkness over the face of the waters" in the book of Genesis. Or maybe, to you, chaos sounds like a preschool, with toddlers running this way and that, squishing playdough into the carpet and sticking their fingers in their ears.

You can think of chaos as something negative, the bits of life that need organizing, that need to be brought under control. Or you can think of chaos as a positive force, as something like raw creativity.

Chaos resists our attempts to define it. It is simply a reality; life itself cannot be neatly predicted. Events spiral out of control. People and situations change. The universe changes.

Chaos can be quite scary, as you contemplate the possibility of everything you know and love as subject to loss, change, and decay. And yet chaos also marks everything as falling into entropy, including the uncomfortable or difficult parts of life. Like the weather, both positive and negative circumstances change. Learning to thrive in the world requires not just coping with change as the fundamental reality but also learning how to shape change in accordance with will. Acknowledging chaos as a basic force allows you to make peace with the whirlwind, and to even use chaos itself as a vehicle to accomplish your deepest desires.

Befriending chaos means courageously going into places of vulnerability and getting into touch with feelings of loss and sadness. As you learn to accept change as a part of all of your experiences, you make room for the positive changes that you would like to see happen.

It does no good to dwell on the past, fixing it in your mind as something ideal and pristine, as we tend to do with fond memories. It also does no good to keep replaying in your mind the negative experiences of years past, which is another way of trying to fix change in place.

In this chapter, you will begin your journey of chaos magick with dedicating your magickal record or grimoire, which you will use throughout this book. You will also create a life map which will help you to identify places and times to practice. You will complete some silent meditations to help declutter your mind for the work to be completed. You will complete a simple spell for seven days of good luck, to get you started on the right path. By the end of this chapter, you will be a working chaos magician, ready to find your own true will and cast it into the universe.

Step 1: Loving the Whirlwind

Befriending chaos means resolutely living in your present reality, however difficult that reality might be. By seeing things as they are, we can begin to think about ways to transcend limitations and find the most rewarding and genuine path.

When we look honestly at ourselves and our lives, we may see quite a lot of mess, even dysfunction. But we can transform the way that we look at that mess and dysfunction, as being full of creative and magickal potential.

The sweet and the bitter go together: we cannot have one without the other. Life contains within it reciprocity and exchange, darkness and light. The opposites define one another. And these qualities blend together ceaselessly in our experiences.

We cannot change this basic complementarity of opposites, but we can move our experiences in one direction or another. By embracing change, we bend reality but also change ourselves in the process. By welcoming chaos, we open ourselves more fully to the world around us and come into our own power as agents of change.

Meditate on these thoughts and seek to love the whirlwind around you.

Step 2: Suspending Your Disbelief

You don't even have to believe in magick to get started as a chaos magician. It is quite normal to have doubts and reservations about whether ritual activity or mental exercises can somehow impact real events. It seems quite impossible for our rationally-minded selves to believe we can affect events outside of our normal cause-and-effect frame of reference. We have been taught to believe that hard work and persistence pay off, that the early bird gets the worm, and other moralistic fables that just so happen to align with the interests of capitalism.

Our society is organized in such a way as to reward a nose-to-the-grindstone mentality, which means that we have a hard time even considering alternative pathways to the fulfillment of desire. It can feel like a costly luxury to engage in magickal practice, because it takes time and resources that are in short supply. It can be hard even to dabble in something, to explore something new, when it doesn't seem like a sure bet.

Give your inner skeptic a seat at the table and a voice in your internal conversation. Just don't let it completely take over. All sorts of things are quite irrational, and yet we still consider them to be real in some sense. Romantic love comes to mind as something impossible to prove or demonstrate like a mathematical equation. And yet the experience of love makes it worthwhile, even if it can be a lot of trouble. Life just wouldn't be the same without it. In the same way, you don't need flowers for your kitchen table: it's just nicer to have them around. And you can survive perfectly well without poetry or music, but your quality of life would be diminished. Therefore, we can allow ourselves little extravagances and eccentricities, like magick, simply because they make life more worthwhile.

The only thing necessary is to suspend disbelief in much the same way as you would when reading a novel or watching a movie. Start by simply doing the practices, and the results will follow in due time. The process will, of course, require a little patience, just like anything else, like learning to bake bread or play the accordion. The first steps will be awkward and faltering. At the outset, it might feel very silly to make a sigil or do a visualization exercise, but don't let that embarrassment stop you.

Growth in life requires making mistakes and sometimes breaking things. It requires persistence in the face of evident defeat. You will have moments of discouragement, but the magick will come if you keep going. I invite you to think that it has already begun, inasmuch as you were willing to pick up this book and give it a try.

Step 3: Dedicating Your Magickal Record

One important tool for chaos magick is the magickal journal, which will serve as a logbook for operations performed. You may also work magick directly through the medium of the journal. It should be regarded not just as a notebook or ledger, but as a living thing with a mind of its own, as a creature and not just as a dead thing.[1]

1 In fact, you should begin to think of all things as alive in some way, as having an aura or life force clinging to them. Magickally charged objects, especially, should be treated with care, as they carry potencies necessary to the work.

To begin, you will need a blank book, lined or unlined, preferably hardbound and designed to lay flat when opened. The book should then be consecrated or dedicated for the purpose of your art.

Think first about what time of day you plan to work your craft. Dedicate the book at the time of day. This doesn't have to be exact: think primarily about either daytime or night.

If the book is to be used during the day, especially for matters pertaining to work, health, and organization, place the book for a few hours in a sunny window or take it outside to the park. Think of the sun's rays as filling the blank pages with energy, cleansing the book of any previous associations.

If the book is to be used at night, or for matters of love, passion, or revenge, give it some exposure to the moon. You can choose an auspicious day, like the full moon for blessing/invocation and the new moon for cursing/banishing.

You need not be exact: think of yourself as crafting a sort of personality for the journal, record, or grimoire that you are making.

Then, take the journal to one of your favorite places, such as a cafe, walking trail, or nature preserve. But do not procrastinate by looking for the perfect locale. Also, if you have a chosen divinity or meditative practice, make sure to center yourself beforehand in the tradition with which you are most familiar.

When you get to your sacred space, anoint the cover of the book with a single drop of essential oil, such as clary sage, eucalyptus, or frankincense. A drop of salt water can be used as a substitute.

Say to yourself some words that seem appropriate, like "I dedicate this book to the great work of transformation" or "I dedicate my craft to the fulfillment of my purpose." Then spend a few minutes visualizing, in as much sensory detail as possible, the aim for which you were drawn to the practice of magick in the first place.

Leave a page or two blank and then go to the first page of your record book. Here it would be good to draw or paste some artwork that fits with the theme of the work that you are going to perform. For new opportunities, you might select an open door or a skeleton key. For love, you could choose a rose or two doves. For money, you could choose some coins or a treasure chest. Pennsylvania Dutch hex signs and quilt patterns also have deep symbolism and can be put to many purposes. Use your intuition here and choose a personally meaningful image. It should evoke your purpose without having to explain it explicitly.

Then, write somewhere on this page your name or initials, along with a motto. For your motto, you could use a favorite quotation or an evocative phrase. If you want to keep your motto secret, use only the first letter of each word. If you can't find a motto, for extra coolness, you can select a Latin one from this list:

abyssus abyssum invocat: deep calleth unto deep

acta non verba: deeds not words

ad altiora tendo: I strive for higher things

ad astra per aspera: to the stars through difficulty

ad victorium: to victory

ars gratia artis: art for the sake of art

carpe noctem: seize the night

fac et spera: do and hope

in nomine diaboli: in the name of the devil

in somnis veritas: in dreams there is truth

memento viveri: remember to live

omnia muntantir, nihil interit: everything changes, nothing perishes

spero meliora: I aspire to greater things

Once you have a piece of artwork and a motto and have sealed the book with your intention, you are ready to go. The only other piece would be to select some music that aligns with your purpose and aesthetic. Play the piece of music several times while you are dedicating your journal, and ingrain it in your own mind as well. Whenever you hear it, the song in question will automatically remind you of your purpose. It is very important to feel the words and music as you hear them and to think of yourself as creating this new being in the form of the book.

Optionally, you can personalize your journal in many additional ways. You may choose a magickal syllable or word that acts as a key to the book. For example, the words of the

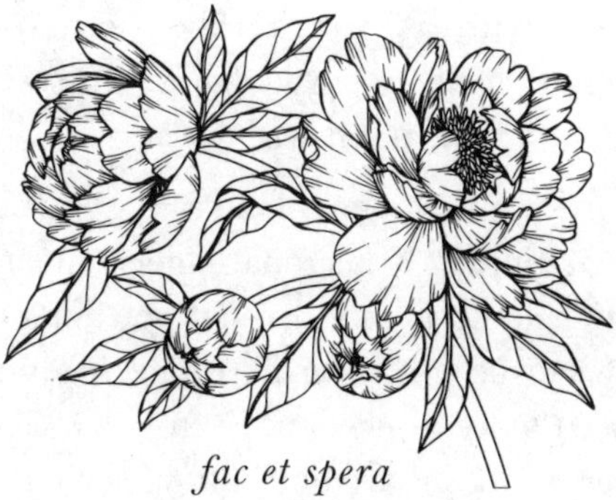

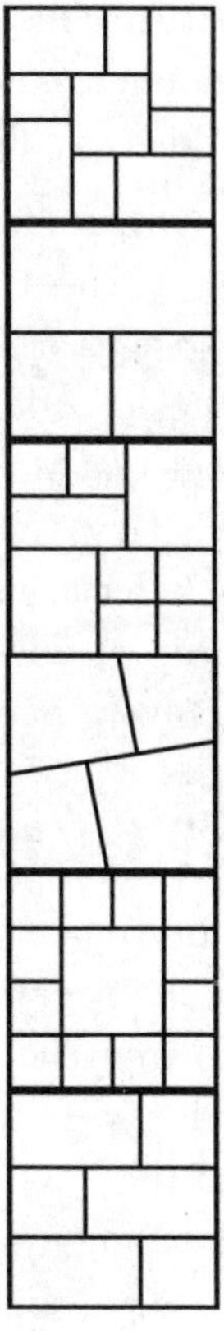

fac et spera

(do and hope)

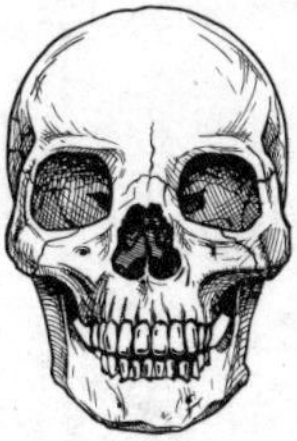

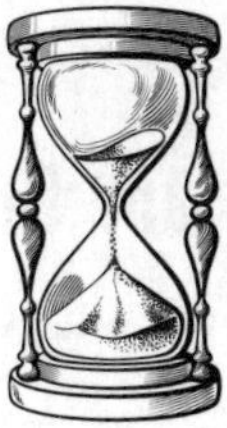

IV. VIII. MMXXV

the dark night of weeping and
wailing will cease.
the soul triumphs over darkening
gloom.
the chains of fear and doubt
disolve.
before the anvil fire of the great
work.

A sample dedication page.

book only work when you pronounce your grandmother's maiden name. Or, if you are familiar with yoga, you could associate the book with a mantra. The words become meaningless except to the person who knows the secret key. Set this as a firm intention, and it will work.

Other measures you can take for secrecy—if that is a concern—are writing in a personal cipher, in multiple languages, or with a numeric code. Even if you don't always write in code, it can be useful to have one ready in the event that you need more discretion. Even if a code is not necessary, you can write in circumlocution, such as using the letter *n.* instead of a person's name. You may also write words of blessing or cursing for the reader, depending upon your purpose for the work.

Step 4: Centering and Grounding

Before undertaking new magickal acts, it is important to ground yourself so that energies may be effectively pushed into your chosen endeavor. Magick across many traditions begins with practices of centering (drawing awareness into the interior of the body-mind nexus) and grounding (becoming aware of the earth and rootedness in place).

These practices of grounding and centering run counter to the impulses of our popular culture, which often propels our attention towards fleeting objects like videos, memes, and listicles. In contrast, centering and grounding require sustained attention.

Cutting back on social media use and internet searches will be a useful way to preserve your focus and mental energy for magickal work. Begin by putting some limits on your internet use, perhaps thirty minutes before noon and thirty minutes in the afternoon. Limiting exposure to advertising is also a beneficial way to gain focus.

Accepting limits just amounts to a grown-up form of self-parenting. We set aside lesser-value activities so we can pursue higher-value activities.

Another good way to retain mental focus is to practice periods of silence, beginning with just ten minutes of silent listening. This can be as simple as setting a timer and sitting quietly, watching your thoughts as they come and go and paying attention to your breath. Once ten minutes comes easily, try moving to fifteen or twenty minutes. This can be done twice a day, once in the morning and once in the evening. Maintaining silence will be a good strengthening exercise for the visualization that comes with magickal practice. Keeping a quiet interior space forms the backdrop for intentional visualization, like a blank canvas for a painter.

Light exercise and generally any form of stress relief also helps maintain concentration during magickal practice.

Step 5: Creating a Life Map

Now that you have consecrated your journal, you will need some regular time to yourself as well as places friendly to your work.

You've already had a taste of this conundrum when you dedicated your magickal record. You may have a schedule that feels too full for ritual work. You may feel that you have no privacy for casting spells without unwanted intrusions. Now is the time to begin finding space and time for yourself.

Ideally, you would have a permanently dedicated ritual space where you could don robes, burn incense, and chant until your heart's content, but very few people have that kind of luxury. And chaos magick is designed to fit into the in-between spaces and times of your life. It does not require idyllic settings or uninterrupted stretches of time. It can be quite nimble and portable.

As a second entry in your magickal record, make a scribble in your journal with a pen or brush. Now look at this scribble and see how messy it is, and note all of the intersections where one line crosses over another. Think of this scribble as a life map to your world. Each intersection represents a point in space and time where you might be able to take a few minutes for your practice.

Now, begin to label the intersections, like, "morning commute in car," "pick up dry cleaning," "9:00 class," "home from work," etc. And note any slight detours that you might make, like "occult bookshop," "explore cemetery," "mirror gazing," etc. You will see very soon that what you thought was a solid block of occupied time is really more like a piece of swiss cheese. You really have spaces throughout your day that you can set aside for the practice, as long as you abandon all notions of doing things perfectly. An abandoned

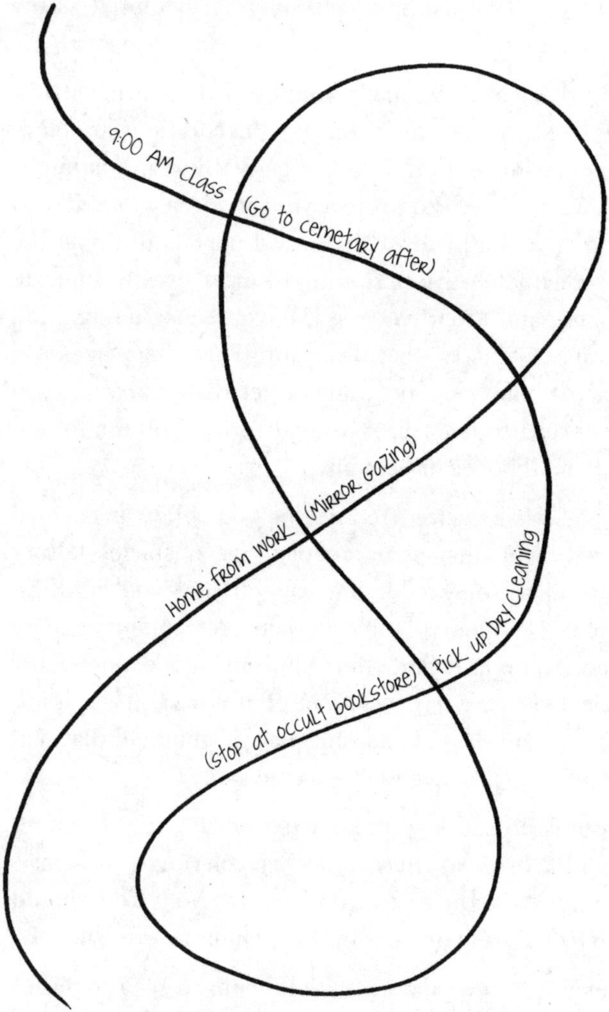

Life map ritual for finding times and places to practice magick

lot in the city has just as much magickal potential as the pyramids at Giza.

Now that you have made your scribble and labeled it, you will want to decorate it. But your decorations are more than just ornamentation. Infuse them with will. You might draw claws and teeth to protect your work from unwanted attention. You might draw doors and portals to invite the help of spiritual entities. You might draw eyes to indicate wakefulness and attentiveness. Use your imagination, and be clear about exactly what you want to have happen as you draw each symbol. If you want to get really creative, you can use thread to embroider your life map. You might add beads or small bones or sequins.

As you work each step, imagine your life transformed into a haven of magickal practice. See obstacles falling away. Visualize yourself living your dreams and fulfilling every goal. Be open to some new images coming to you unbidden. You might find yourself drawing a dandelion or a thimble. Don't try to make sense of it now: you are doing a lot of work on the unconscious part of yourself that will connect to your practice in unexpected ways.

There is no set way of knowing when you are "done" with your life map. You may stop when you run out of space, or it may just begin to feel finished for you. You should begin to feel a sense of possibility opening in your life.

Over the coming days, you will begin to see the places you frequent with new eyes. You will see connections you hadn't noticed before, and you will begin to make small adjustments that make your life much more amenable to the practice. Most importantly, you will begin to discover some breathing room that you didn't know that you had—spaces in your life that you can keep to your intuitive, creative self.

You can repeat this ritual at intervals throughout your practice: maybe once per season or whenever you experience life or schedule changes. For example, moving to a new home is a massive recalibration that this ritual can ease.

Step 6: Giving Yourself Rest

Sometimes the best thing you can do for your practice is to know when to rest. Think of the rests in a piece of music. Those pauses make the rhythm possible. They can be short jots or full stops, breathing breaks or profound silences. They are just as much a part of the musical piece as the notes themselves.

And as you practice your craft, you will have off days when it feels like you have not accomplished anything. Life gets in the way. The pipes in the house burst. Work demands more of you than usual. You catch a cold, or some chronic health problem gets in the way. On some days, you will do well to just make a cup of tea and take a nap. Taking pauses is part of the work. The so-called interruptions are part of the transformation. Remember that chaos magick works on life itself, through the medium of life as it is.

Work in a push-and-pull with life. You don't want to "go with the flow" so much that you become completely passive, and you also don't want to be so rigid that you lose perspective. Look for the skillful interventions that will improve your life. Find the efficiencies and use the moments that you have been given.

You will develop an inner sense for when you are feeling strong: you will have powerful intuitions about the next steps to take in your practice, and synchronicities will bring you needed resources with little effort.

When you are not feeling strong magickally, you may have feelings of defeatism, and skeptical doubts may seem overwhelming. It might seem like nothing is working right.

In order to maintain inner strength and resolve, you will need to feel well, mentally and physically. A regimen of light exercise, such as walking or jogging, will be beneficial, as will getting a good night's sleep.

Meditation should be practiced as often as possible. There are endless variations of meditative practice from around the world, but the simplest way to meditate is to sit silently and listen to whatever arises for you. Allow the thoughts and emotions to come and go as they will. Do this for ten minutes a day to start.

Later in this book, we will get into some more complex forms of meditation and visualization. Just keep in mind that more complex does not mean more advanced. Silence is the best teacher, and the more you can expose yourself to quiet solitude, the more rapidly you will progress. Interior silence will be more valuable than sitting in a quiet room. With practice, you will be able to sit next to a busy intersection or in a crowded train station with a quiet mind and heart.

At times of major emotional upset, such as during a breakup or after the death of a loved one, be extra gentle with yourself. Make sure to use meditation as a way to acknowledge strong emotions and not flee from them. Don't attempt to use spiritual means to short-circuit the natural grieving process. Also, there is no need to force yourself to complete a ritual if you do not feel up to it. The magick will be there for you when you are ready for it.

It is okay to allow yourself time to do nothing at all, as much as your life will allow. The lifelong transformation process of magickal consciousness gives us more ease and peace, but it does so over years and decades. Knowing that truth deep down will take away some of the desire for quick results.

Step 7: Seven Days of Good Luck

To begin your magickal journey with chaos magick, set your intentions for one week of good luck. Our use of the seven-day week traces back to the ancient Babylonians, who had star charts dating back thousands of years before the Greeks. They derived the number seven from the seven bodies they viewed in the night sky: the sun, the moon, Mercury, Venus, Mars, Jupiter, and Saturn.

These bodies come to us via successive layers of cultural significance, through the Greeks and the Romans. Each week is another chance for us to build on these celestial influences and to make something great of the lifetime that each of us has been given. From the sun, we gain inspiration and the ability to lead. Through the moon, we practice devotion and gain intuition. Mercury teaches skill in communication and yields intellectual insight. Venus yields sensitivity to beauty and gives access to love. Mars allows self-assertion and courage. Jupiter imparts wisdom and authority. Saturn yields self-discipline and perseverance. We need all of these qualities to live a good life, and correctly balancing them leads to a lucky life.

Begin your week-long blessing by drawing seven points on a blank page in your magickal record. These seven points will represent the seven days in the week to come, beginning the day after you perform this exercise. Once you have drawn the points, connect them together with lines. You may get a perfect seven-pointed star, or you may get something lopsided—it matters not at all. Then, for each day of the week, write your true wish for that day in only one word. The thing that matters most here is sincerity: do not wish for world peace if you truly desire sex and money. Lack of firmness in purpose will distort the results. (If you wish to avoid prying eyes, write in runes or in cipher.)

Next, randomly assign a cosmic body to each day of the week. For this process, use a random number generator, easily available on the internet. You will assign the numbers as follows: 1 = the sun, 2 = the moon, 3 = Mercury, 4 = Venus, 5 = Mars, 6 = Jupiter, 7 = Saturn. (They may also be assigned randomly.) Note that one body may come up more than once, while others may not come up at all. This may indicate that you need more practice with a particular planetary energy, while you may be stronger in other areas.

You will now have a particular wish for each day, combined with a celestial energy to serve as the focus for that day. As each day dawns, say a few words to invoke that body. For example, for the sun you might say, "I invite the rays of the sun, bringer of inspiration and leadership. May my day be blessed with heat and life." Then spend five to ten minutes meditating on that celestial body sometime in the morning, preferably first thing.

Then, as you go throughout the day, make sure to record in your magickal journal any blessings you gained that day as you focused on making your life more fruitful and enjoyable. Above all, know in your heart and mind that things will improve as you concentrate your will on increasing your luck for the span of seven days. If you forget to say your invocation for a day, do not worry. Simply continue the next day as planned. With exercises like this, you gradually build your concentration and willpower for the rituals to come.

If you have trouble tapping into the energy of a particular cosmic body, try looking at artwork associated with it, which may also be considered a deity in various different cultures.It also helps to read historic invocations and poetry pertaining to that celestial body or deity.

Copy down any relevant quotations into your magickal record, but only if that fragment of literature really speaks to you. Rote memorization generally will not help you to capture the vibration of the body in question, the factor most necessary for the success of the work. Once you have acquainted yourself with that cosmic body, it will become much easier to perform the invocation in the future, like stopping at the house of an old friend.

As you go through the week, meditating on each celestial body, take note of any good things that come your way during that week as a result of the meditation. For example, perhaps you were meditating on Venus and an artist friend gave you a painting to hang in your home. Or perhaps working with Mercury helped you to finish a big writing project. Maybe working with Mars helped you confront an overbearing supervisor or a shady landlord. By taking note of these blessings flowing into your life, you befriend the planets, moon, and sun and make it easier for you to work with them in the future.

Many Roads, Many Doors

This book will open many pathways for self-understanding, spiritual growth, and life transformation. By choosing the path of chaos magic, you step outside of conventional belief systems, in which one right way trumps all others. You choose instead a way of life where many roads converge and where many doors can be opened. Some of those doors lead deeper into your own subconscious mind, while others lead to other planes of existence.

Instead of choosing just one system and one way, you open yourself to the wisdom of the ages from the traditions of the world. You didn't just stumble across the chaos path:

you have been walking these many roads for years. You will find much here that feels warm and familiar, and this is a sign that you are finding your true calling as a spiritual being and magickal practitioner.

Take this opportunity to make a simple vow to yourself, that you will give yourself the gift of the exercises in this book, and that you will be as generous with your time and resources as your life will allow. Vow to finish the chapters in this book and to continue to create your own magickal record, so that this time in your life will be filled with enchantment.

When you realize you have stepped closer to your true self and full potential, you will be able to look back on this time with a smile.

May your inner light grow ever brighter and all obstacles be removed as you undertake this journey to your true self.

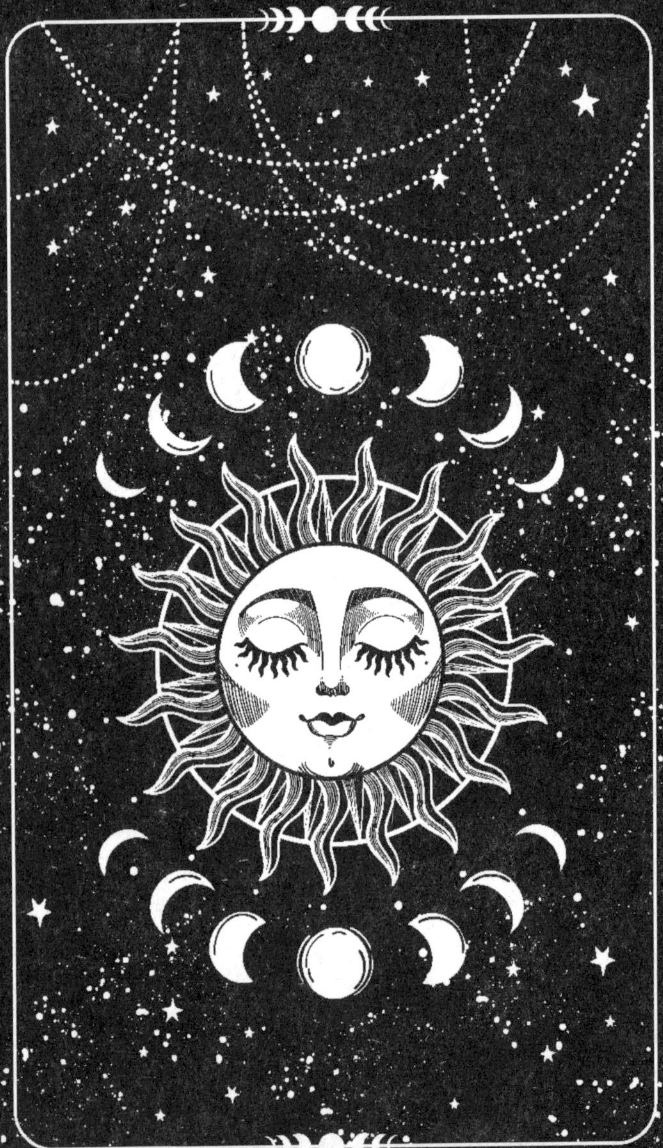

Chapter 2: Diving Deeper into Chaos Magick

In this chapter, you will continue your journey of chaos magick with two meditations that will be useful in all of the other spells to come. You will learn to visualize the chaosphere, a cube inscribed within a sphere with lines radiating in all directions, a sacred shape that represents potential becoming actual. You will also learn the qabalistic cross meditation, a ritual that has both empowering and protective functions. And you will also complete the sacred spiral ritual, which will give you insight into the state of your relationships and provide you with ways to optimize these relationships for your success. By the end of this chapter, you will have many new techniques for getting in touch with your true self and for projecting your desire into the universe.

In the last chapter, you learned to use some tools that inaugurate the process of chaos magick. You dedicated or awakened your magickal record that holds self-created esoteric lore. You vowed to persevere in this pursuit at least until the end of this book, if not for a lifetime. Take a moment to appreciate what you have done so far. These tools may seem simple, but, when applied over time, they land you in a much different, more satisfying place than the way of complacency and apathy.

Moving forward, make sure to open your magickal record at least once per day. Start a heading with the time and date. Record how you are feeling, mentally and physically. If you like, record the weather and astrological conditions. Then make note of any exercises performed and the results that you experienced. Be prepared for spontaneous occurrences: your practice will lead to sudden insights into life situations that had baffled you before. You may see your relationships, your work, your finances in a new light. Record these new understandings and be prepared to act on them.

Now that some of the basic practices are in place, we will begin to expand on them through slightly more difficult exercises. Remember that, if you feel lost, you can always return to previous chapters. It is more important to do a few things well than to do a lot of things badly. So take your time, stay grounded, and remember to practice self-care as discussed in the previous chapter. Go at the pace your life allows. Do not neglect your everyday duties for the sake of magic, as any neglect will lead to harsh karma. At the same time, do not be afraid to begin: your practice expands the moment you say yes to it.

Step 1: Understanding the Higher Self and the Astral Body

Writers like Peter J. Carroll and Phil Hine revived chaos magick in the 1990s in order to synthesize older traditions of ceremonial magick with aspects of witchcraft and neopaganism, along with an explicit appeal to science and pop culture. Chaos acted as a kind of glue holding together disparate strands of thought with a kind of rebellious ethos and eclectic borrowing. This chapter will take aspects of this earlier generation's work and make it more relevant for today's LGBTQIA+ magicians.

Chaos plays the part of a great goddess, reminiscent of the role of Maya in Hinduism and Buddhism or the unceasing change of Heraclitus in the west. Chaos has an aspect of primordial power, that which lies beyond rational thought, and yet simultaneously relates to the play of appearances that animate our lives. Chaos speaks to the unceasing tendency towards change that characterizes life in the world: in vain do we try to resist it. Rather, the only power available to humanity lies in acknowledging and befriending chaos, fusing the individual will with the greater will of nature.

The magician strives to access the dream or astral body, which can be used for magickal journeys and undertakings. But the astral body is powerless without a connection to the higher soul or self. The higher self cannot be perceived directly, but its awakening can be felt with feelings of bliss as well as a heightened sense of genius or inspiration in taking action. The meditations in this chapter will deepen your connection to the higher self or inner genius. as unlocking the astral body or inner senses will become the basis for magickal work.

The higher self remains unseen and invisible, divine in nature, serene and controlled. It is the abiding center we find in quiet contemplation. The dream body or astral body, by contrast, is one of the subtle bodies, the body we use in dreams and visualization. Magick happens when we link the higher self to the dream body in alignment with will. The exercises that follow will enable this connection.

Peter J. Carroll writes, "Every moment the consortium of 'I' puts on a new face. I am not who I was a few seconds ago, much less yesterday. Our name is multiple. I am a colony of beings sharing the same envelope."

The moment you close your eyes to meditate, you hear not one but a cacophony of voices. Chaos magick does not seek to blunt or badger the discord into harmony, but to simply attend to the inner tumult and work with it. The higher self or inner genius does not speak above the din, but rather within and through it.

Step 2: The Chaosphere

The chaosphere is a mystical shape described by Peter J. Carroll in *Liber Null* that has precursors in the Golden Dawn system of ceremonial magick and in the texts of Thelema, the magickal system inaugurated by Aleister and Rose Crowley in the Cairo Working of 1904. This mystical shape is full of deep symbolism, and it also has practical uses that will be explored here.

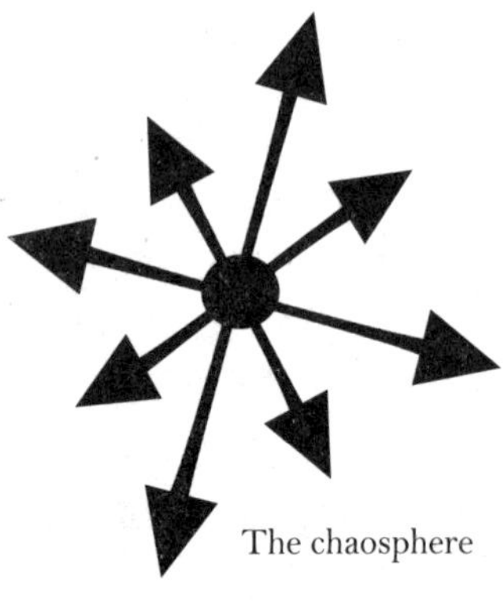

The chaosphere

The chaosphere is a way of making the formless void

comprehensible to the mind. The shape is described as a cube inscribed inside of a sphere, with arrows radiating toward the eight vertices of the cube. The sphere contains the contradictory forces of light and darkness and all other contraries as well, in its inherently paradoxical nature. The cube and sphere may take physical form as a fetish object in the temple, but its primary nature is etheric or astral. What follows is a simple meditation to access the chaosphere.

Set a timer for ten minutes. Sit in a chair with eyes closed, spine straight, head level, feet shoulder-width apart. Hands should be placed on the thighs, palms down, gently resting. Take six "box breaths": breathing in four counts, holding for four counts, exhaling four counts, holding four counts.

After this cycle has been repeated six times, visualize a transparent sphere of blue-white light above the head. The light becomes more intense and illuminates the interior darkness, driving out extraneous thoughts and impulses. The sphere stabilizes and expands to the size of a beach ball and rotates above the head of the aspirant.[2] A cube appears inside the sphere, each corner perfectly intersecting the curve. Next, eight arrows emerge from the center of the sphere, each intersecting one corner of the cube.

---

2 By *aspirant*, I simply mean someone who wants to do this type of magick and receive results from it. Chaos magick has no centralized authority, although there are organized orders such as the Illuminates of Thanateros (IoT). Thee Temple of Psychick Youth (TOPY, see below) fractured in the early 1990s.

Let the magician fix this image as closely as possible. Then, allow the chaosphere to rotate in the mental space, each of its features glowing in blue-white light.

Call to mind the following reflection: *I dissolve my thoughts into the blue-white light of chaos. I release my thoughts into the All. I dissolve my feelings into the blue-white light of chaos. I release my feelings into the All. I dissolve my actions into the blue-white light of chaos. I release my actions into the All. I have become indifferent to gain and loss. I have become indifferent to pain and pleasure. All roads converge for me in the All. My dream is my destiny and mine alone. I have become chaos, progenitor and destroyer of worlds.*

Close the meditation by picturing the chaosphere moving down the axis of the body, from above the head (*sahāsrara*) to between the eyes (*ajña*) to the heart (*anahāta*).[3] The blue-white light then suffuses the entire body, cleansing the body and spirit of toxic habitualities. You may, upon close of the ritual, make a mental intention for the day.

This meditation is best repeated three times per day, especially before sleep. With repeated practice of thirty days or more, you will be able to form the chaosphere in sleep. The chaosphere may be used for astral travel, to neutralize psychic threats, or to begin new initiatives. Place your desire at the center of the sphere and see the eight rays

---

3 The *sahāsrara*, literally "thousand petalled," chakra resides at the crown of the head and is said to resemble an inverted lotus. *Ajña* means "to command or perceive," and meditating on this point gives increased concentration and insight. *An hata*, the heart chakra, means "unstruck" or "unwounded." Its presence may be encountered in a ringing sound heard during meditation.

projecting that desire throughout the universe. You will then receive synchronic hints and suggestions throughout the day that lead to fulfillment of desire.

Make sure to write down the results of this meditation in your magickal record.

Step 3: The Chaosphere and Your True Will

Within the chaosphere, the sphere represents pure potential, while the cube represents possibility taking concrete form. The many arrows radiating from the center of the cube show that many possibilities remain open to us in any given moment, and yet we must freely choose among those possibilities as we work to unfold our desired future. The process of choosing is the possible becoming actual. And as magicians, we seek to unfold our highest will, the best and most true of the possibilities open to us. The law of Crowley's Thelema, "Do what thou wilt shall be the whole of the law," has its counterpart in the Wiccan rede, "An' it harm none, do what ye will."

In the coming days, months, and years, in what ways do you want your creativity to manifest itself? Spend some time writing in your magickal journal about it. Maybe you have always wanted to write a one-act play, learn to do pottery, or hike the Appalachian trail. Maybe you want to find a new lover, get a tattoo, or visit Nepal.

Have the courage and boldness to write about your emerging idea. Set up a heading in your journal that says something like, "What I Want to Have Happen." Then, freewrite for ten to twenty minutes about what you want to occur over the coming year or so. Use vivid sensory details. Infuse your writing with holy will—the feeling and energy that your vision will become true.

Once you have clarified your vision, think of possible obstacles to the manifestation of your will. Maybe you will need some additional money or time off work. Maybe you haven't met the right client or the right partner to make your vision a reality. Maybe you face self-doubt or a gap in skills that you think will make the project difficult. Just jot down a brief list of obstacles to your vision.

Then, without missing a beat, write down a few words about how you will counter each obstacle. So, for example, if you need to learn a new software program, you might take a course online to make up for the missing knowledge.

Close your journaling practice with a deep feeling that you will make your vision come true. In a future chapter, you will learn how to make sigils to help you manifest your will. For now, just know that whatever you wrote will become a reality for you. But you will have to exercise maximal effort, both in your magickal practice and in your everyday work.

One small caveat: you should feel an electric current of energy move through your body when you record your true will. Your goal should be at least a little bit thrilling, a little bit subversive even. If your heart doesn't skip a beat, you may be setting a goal that doesn't really spark your enthusiasm. In that case, what you have is more of a to-do list than a genuine statement of will.

Your goal should not feel impossible, but it should not be easy, either. It should feel just beyond the reach of your current abilities, and it should require at least some resources, like time, money, and energy, that you do not currently have.

Over the coming weeks, as you move through this book and create your magickal record, you will demonstrate that you can make difficult things happen, even things that seem impossible to you now. You are following a path of tremendous growth that will move you forward, due to the awakening of and expression of your true will.

Step 4: Exploring the Chaosphere

After working with the chaosphere several times, you will note that you can make the sphere as large or small as you would like in your mind's eye. In the beginning, you practiced envisioning it in the space above your head. Perhaps you pictured it as being about a foot in diameter.

This time, use all of the same preliminaries as in the earlier meditation, but try making the chaosphere much larger, so that you can fit your entire body inside. You should see yourself at the center of a cube circumscribed by a sphere, with eight rays going out toward the corners of the cube. The four walls of the cube now correspond to the four cardinal directions, and the eight corners to the half directions. By invoking the chaosphere, you have a way of consecrating your ritual space that can be used for any magickal operation.

Whether you cast the chaosphere while sitting or standing, you now have at your feet a crossroads, with the four paths going in the four cardinal directions. The crossroads is a traditional place of meeting for processes of magickal exchange.

At this time, you may wish to get into contact with your guardian angel or higher genius. You may wish to commune with the deities or orishas of any given pantheon—African, Indic, Norse, Greek, Egyptian, etc. You may want to contact Hekate, goddess of boundaries, or Lucifer, the prince of the Craft. Each deity or spirit will have certain procedures, hymns, offerings, etc., proper to the tradition to which they belong.

You may also improvise your own rites and rituals using what you know of the entity to be invoked. Casting the chaosphere ahead of time puts you into the proper frame of mind, so that you can become more open to the experience. It also serves as a sort of portable temple when you don't have the ability to find a perfect setting. Additionally, you don't really need to "power down" the chaosphere or have a formal closing—as soon as your mind begins to wander to mundane things, the chaosphere tends to easily dissolve.

Chaosphere meditation also produces the effect of tranquility in various life circumstances, as any outcome can be viewed as a manifestation of chaos. If you experience good fortune, that experience contains within it the flipside of poverty and lack. Whether your stomach is full or empty, these contrarities are simple inversions of one another. In short, by repeated meditation on chaos, you gradually lose aversion for circumstances perceived as negative or loathsome.

At first, chaosphere meditation may lead to erratic swings of emotion or behavior. And yet these swings also amount to the deliberate practice of randomness, injecting spontaneity into rigid worldviews and conditioned behaviors. You may soon find new pathways of action where once the way seemed impenetrable. Because, while the chaosphere can be viewed as a symbol of destruction, it also brings about growth in the wake of that destruction. Chaos has a devouring, consuming aspect that hews away disused beliefs. When this mental and spiritual detritus has been cleared away, new growth can occur in earnest.

The arrows of the chaosphere point in opposite directions, showing that every belief, thought, and action has its contrary pole. With every attitude or belief, imagine what it would be like to believe exactly the opposite. Practice arguing with yourself, testing your beliefs to see if they hold muster.

Maybe you have some pop psychological beliefs about yourself. Maybe you think you are too selfish when you actually are too accommodating. Maybe you think you are codependent when you actually try to go it alone too often.

No matter what, allow the chaosphere to sift your thoughts and beliefs, and even allow you to practice random beliefs. For example, you could try espousing a different religion for a few weeks. Argue for different points of view, at least as an exercise.

This will give you insight into other people and into yourself. You may find yourself learning more about the world than you would have by staying in a rut. Most of your experiments with different truths will not last, but that is okay—the point is to see that disparate belief systems can simultaneously be true, each in their own way and on their own terms.

Step 5: The Qabalistic Cross

The qabalistic cross meditation powerfully recharges the energetic body (*prānamāya kosha*)[4] with a minimal use of time and concentration. It can also be conducted nearly anywhere in a discrete fashion, making it ideal for use in our hectic times. Most people know the qabalistic cross as the opener for the Lesser Banishing Ritual of the Pentagram, but it is a valuable piece of magick in its own right, not to be hurried or neglected. Try repeating the following meditation three times per day for maximum effect.

Begin with the box breath that you used for the chaosphere meditation. Then, let go of counting breath and visualize the night sky all around. The Earth comes to seem like a small speck situated at the feet of your astral body.

Visualize a disk of powerful light situated just above the head, at the *sahāsrāra* chakra. The orb of light sends a

4 *Kosha* means sheath, and the physical body amounts to only one layer of several bodies. *Pr na* is a subtle cosmic energy that moves throughout the universe, but it can be directed into the body through meditation and breathwork.

ray downward into the *ajña* chakra between the eyes, where a second orb of bright light radiates.

Intone the syllables *ATAH* ("Thou art") into the space between the eyes.

The light proceeds downward into the chest region, where you will vibrate the divine name *HERU-RA-HA*, with a mighty explosion of light emanating from your chest at the *anahāta* chakra.

At your feet, intone, *MALKOOT*, the name of the foundation sephirah, with a similar sphere of light radiating there.

From malkuth, attention shifts to the right shoulder, where the words *VEH-GEBURAH* ("Thine be the power") are vibrated in a sphere of light.

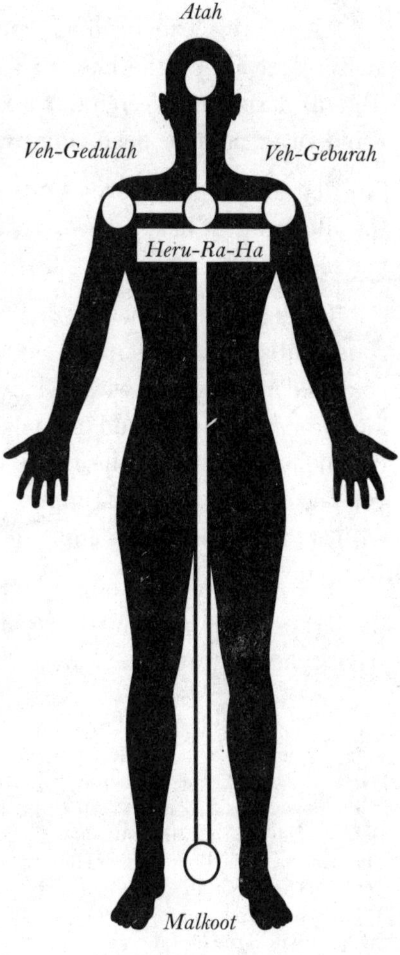

The qabalistic cross

Similarly, at the left shoulder, intone, *VEH-GEDULAH* ("And the glory").

Finally, closing at the chest, pronounce, *LEH-OLAHM* ("Forever and ever").[5]

All of this can be done mentally, with no outward gestures at all, or the magician may use the ficus mudra (thumb clasped between index and middle finger in a fist), a wand, or an athame, gesturing towards each sephirah.[6]

Repeat this procedure as many times as necessary until the allotted time has expired, perhaps ten to fifteen minutes per session.

The lights of the qabalistic cross form a sort of internal constellation of great power. Once the lights have been activated and charged with the divine names, they become a focus for meditation. You can take the stance of adoration, in which the light is of the divine, or of absorption, in which you become one with that light. Most likely, you will begin with adoration and move more deeply into absorption.

The above names should be repeated many times, and the lights made to glow as brightly as possible. With each repetition, the feeling or *bhava* of divinity grows stronger.

---

5 Sometimes the qabalistic cross exercise is viewed simply as the preamble to the Lesser Banishing Ritual of the Pentagram (LBRP), but it is a powerful ritual in its own right. In fact, the full LBRP will not yield its fruit if the qabalistic cross is performed in a careless manner. The names invoked here are in Hebrew, except for *Heru-ra-ha*, which is Crowley's term for an emanation of Horus, signifying the inner divinity

6 The *sephirot* (singular, *sephirah*) are the ten nodes of divine energy on the qabalistic Tree of Life.

Gradually, you will become capable of doing the meditation constantly, even while engaged in other tasks. You will become more tolerant of noisy, crowded conditions while still concentrating on the sephirah. In this way, the qabalistic cross becomes a refuge from unfavorable conditions and a shield from psychic attack. It sharpens the will and increases the power of mundane and magickal work alike. It is an important path opener that shows the way to greater self-understanding and deep intuition.

In this meditation, six is an important number. Correlated to the chaosphere, the six phrases in the qabalistic cross exercise correlate to the six sides of the cube of Hadit inside the sphere of Nuit. Thinking about this cube as a six-sided die, you can see that Hadit represents possibility, all of the various outcomes coming to fruition. Repeated thrice, six is also the number of the beast, the proclaimer of the new aeon of Horus the child, as well as Satan or Lucifer, the bringer of light and knowledge. Six is also said to be the number of the heart, responsible for deep feelings of universal love and respect. It is also a symbol of creativity, with oversight for artistic production.

Step 6: Chaos, Gender, and Sexuality

The chaosphere suggests that nothing has a fixed essence, and this connects directly to queerness: people are fluid entities in their sexual proclivities and gender expressions. You can be attracted to men, women, nonbinary people, or any combination thereof. You can feel super masc one day and a bit femme three hours later. It is okay to put on different outfits, different costumes, different identities, from one day to the next. Gender is a masquerade, to be enjoyed from various angles and perspectives, at different times and seasons of life.

Think about some of the gay bars you have visited. Maybe you think of a concrete block building by the side of the railroad tracks, neon sign out front, a huge pride flag displayed prominently. The drinks are cheap and never-ending. Think about how the various subcultures coexist awkwardly there—lesbians, nonbinary people, drag queens and kings, gay men, bisexual and bicurious people, etc. Within these four gin-soaked walls, the straight continuum breaks in half, and there lies everything that does not belong in the straight world. This kind of cacophony of queerness represents humanity itself—vibrant, diverse, and changeable.

The chaosphere holds all of these possible identities, both separately and as alterations of one another. As you meditate on the chaosphere, you might think about your gender and sexual identity, not just in general, but today, this morning, or this afternoon. Whether you came out yesterday or decades ago, your individual expression matters, and it matters that you feel in touch with yourself as you are right now. This self-knowledge closely connects with fantasy, both in terms of who you would like to be and who you would like to be with. Allow the chaosphere to take you there, to the place where you feel most yourself and most attracted to that special someone.

As you do the chaosphere meditation or the qabalistic cross, think about this ritual as scouring away predetermined expectations for who you can become. You don't have to abide by the expectations that your parents set for you as a young person or by society's expectations for you now. You don't even have to be bound by what you felt a day or two ago. You are free to choose how you will dress, how you will wear your hair, and whether or not to wear makeup. You can choose infinite costumes and accessories. How you present yourself will be up to you.

Above all, play around! Experiment! Chaos magick came into your life at this moment, because you were looking for fresh air. As a result of doing these practices, you will find yourself having intuitions and hunches. These hunches could be very vague, like you just know you want to dress a little more sophisticated or a little more punk rock. Or you might receive more precise guidance, like the desire for a handknit wool sweater or an emerald brooch. When these urges come to you, do your best to fulfill them. You will feel better as a result of following your inner intuition.

Intuition comes in many different forms. You may feel attracted to a new restaurant or a new club. You may find yourself attracted to someone who isn't your "type." You may crave new foods that didn't previously whet your palette. You may delve into new forms of art and literature.

The chaos engine opens you to all sorts of new influences and daydreams. Don't neglect any of them, because you never know how the change you want to create will enter your life. Remember that chaos works in a nonlinear fashion to give you your heart's desire.

Step 7: The Sacred Spiral

Begin a new page in your magickal record or select a sheet of art paper. You will also need a pen and either liquid ink or liquid paint, such as diluted watercolor or acrylic paint.

Burn some incense with the intention of removing distraction and negativity. Center using the chaosphere or the qabalistic cross.

Begin by drawing a spiral on your paper, starting in the center of the page and working your way outward. Make sure to fill the entire page with this spiral. Around the edges, you will have some uncompleted loops, and that will be just fine. Do not worry about making your spiral perfect.

Next, take some diluted paint or ink and splatter it on the page using a wet brush. You might also use a dropper bottle if the splatter technique sounds too messy. You can stop here, if you like, or do another round or two, perhaps with a different color.

The spiral here represents yourself, with the center of the spiral standing for your heart or soul. The outer rings of the spiral stand for the more surface aspects of your personality, the self or selves that you present to the world. The blotches of ink or paint that you splattered represent the other people in your life. You can now begin to interpret the ink splotches intuitively. Ink splotches near the center mean you have people close to your heart, while a lot of peripheral splotches means you can be defensive and have a hard time letting people into your confidence.

From here, you can get more artful with your interpretation. By all means, develop your own system, but a few general rules apply. Love relationships generally come from the upper right quadrant, while career-related influences come from the bottom center and bottom right. Relationships pertaining to wealth reside in the upper left quadrant, while health-related influences come from the left center. Generally, the interpretation follows a feng shui bagua map, if you would like to pull one up on your computer. By reading the spiral, you will gain a good understanding of where your relationships stand at the present time, as well as where you tend to place your time and attention.

To use the spiral as a spell, simply add paint splotches where you would like them to be. For example, to attract a life mate, place a dot near the center of the upper right quadrant. For more of a casual relationship, place it a bit further from the heart center. To attract friendship, use the lower right quadrant. Burn a candle with the light shed on your spiral while envisioning the outcome you desire. Gaze upon the spiral for a few minutes each night before bed for one waxing moon cycle, from new to full. At the end of this period, you will be able to repeat the exercise to see how things have shifted.

Step 8: Developing Proper Confidence

You can make progress on the magickal path with enough perseverance and self-understanding. Each of us has innate divinity that can be hidden but not effaced completely. We all go through seasons of doubt and fear in which we feel unsure of ourselves and our place in the world. Know that you can move forward even in the most difficult of times, because your heart of hearts will be there to provide you with solace and comfort, guidance and inspiration.

You might find yourself carried away at times by the prospects of the magickal arts for attracting love and wealth into your life. Most people do have some extrinsic motivation in mind when they begin to study magic. But the real secret lies in your true nature, which is already one with God, the universe, or the All. It is best not to get bogged down in theological controversy or using the correct terminology. Just think of yourself, deep within, beneath the personality and memory, as infinitely good and wise.

You may imagine this deep, inward self as like a wise grandparent or a spontaneous young child. After sitting for some time in silence, you might engage in conversation with this inner guide. You can bring your questions, your heartaches, your problems to this wiser self within the self, and you will receive answers when you ask with belief. Only be prepared to have your frame of reference shifted and your perspective broadened: by talking to your inner guide, you are doing nothing less than communing with all of existence.

The true work of magick, the genuine inner alchemy, is all about strengthening your connection with your inmost self. As this connection grows stronger, you will be able to consult your inner guide or higher genius throughout the day. Intuition will guide you, and serendipity will grace your path. While you will still have problems in life, you will obsess over them less and find solutions more smoothly. You will experience a lack of concern with mundane details as they simply fall into place.

An Ongoing Invitation

As you move deeper into this book and craft your own magickal record, you may be tempted at times to abandon the practice altogether. There will be a voice within your head that tells you that you are a grown-up and that it is time to "put away childish things," like believing in magick. During these times, it will seem entirely impractical to do your meditations and exercises. And you do, in fact, have responsibilities that need your attention, but you are not a machine made only for work. If you take time for magick, for spirit, for the things of the heart, you will be protected by your craft.

Over the coming days and weeks, your life will subtly invite you to spend time on your journey of chaos magic. Perhaps, on your way to work, you notice a used bookstore where an interesting tome waits. Maybe you find a spare half hour to sit in meditation. Maybe you receive hidden guidance when the hair stands up on the back of your neck.

You may find yourself inventing your own pathways of magick as your intuition grows. You may outwardly do the exact same things in your life, but behind the scenes, your strength and resolve grows. Confidence builds in your heart as you intone the aforementioned divine names and contact your inner genius.

Take this time to congratulate yourself on your progress thus far. Make note of any interesting occurrences and any intuitions that have come to you as a result of this practice. If you feel moved, share your experiences with a friend in the queer community, online or in real life. There may be others out there who would benefit from your insight. Then, take a day or two of rest to prepare yourself for the adventure ahead.

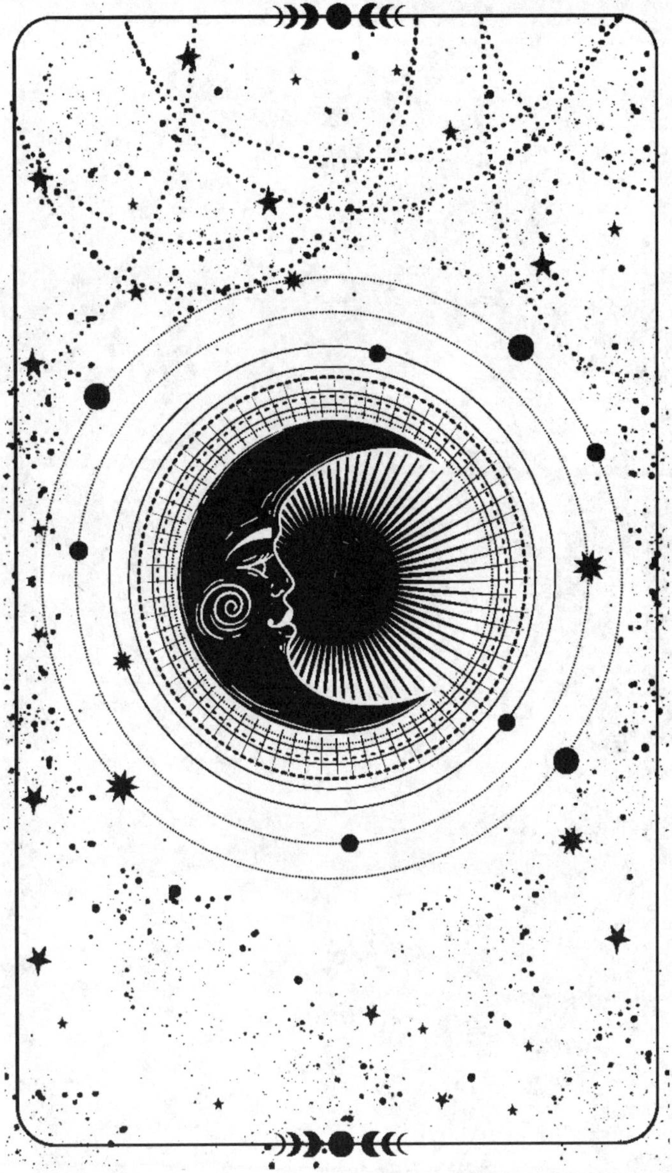

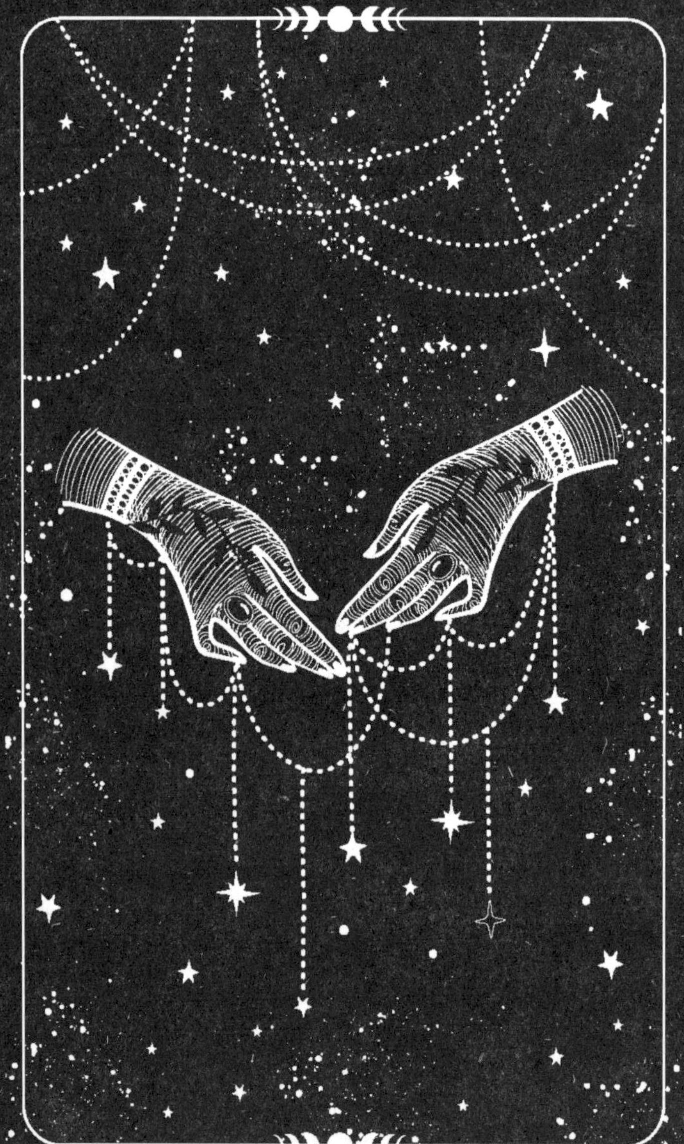

Chapter 3: Chaos Sigil Magick

In this chapter, you will learn how to construct a sigil, a magickal tool that will empower any project you consider to be worthy of your time and attention. You will gain greater peace and clarity in your life as you learn to focus on a goal and devote psychic resources toward it.

Each phase of the sigil-creation process will be described in detail, from idea to realization.

As you step into the sigil creation process, remember this: chaos can destroy our preconceptions, but it can also give life in the form of new avenues of possibility. It undermines everything, and yet it is the matrix-mother-womb that allows for all of experience to arise. Each and every day we live within chaos, and our comfort with this primal reality determines the depth of our will to live. A strong will toward life provides a way to navigate the maelstrom, to cross the abyss and find our true selves.

In the previous chapter, you discovered some new tools for finding and expressing your true self. You awakened the energetic and astral bodies through the qabalistic cross exercise and the chaosphere meditation. You came into greater touch with your own queerness and learned to transform your relationships with the sacred spiral. You are learning to cross the abyss with some powerful tools at your disposal, tools that help you to feel grounded and connected in the midst of an ever-changing world.

In this chapter, your magickal practice is beginning to crest like a wave. You have now reached the point where you can create magickal sigils to help you accomplish your heart's desire. This chapter will guide you through the sigil creation process, from idea to manifestation. This will be a chance to let your creativity shine and to sharpen your magickal will.

Step 1: Finding Your Materials

This chapter introduces sigil creation using the cut-up technique, which involves writing something in prose, cutting the writing into pieces, and then re-assembling it.

The results? Surprising juxtapositions and revelatory turns of phrase.

Key phrases from the cut-up can then be incorporated into a sigil, which will be a central text augmented with artwork. The artwork may be original paintings and drawings, or simply photos clipped from a magazine and arranged into a collage.

The process works, but it also *worlds,* in the sense of making new things possible. Art, magick and spirituality amount to one and the same thing—the manipulation of materials to evoke inner and outer change.

You will work on finding magick in plain sight, using everyday materials. There are gates of access, portals to entry, on every street corner and in every newspaper.

As a starting assignment, be on the lookout for images and texts that speak to you. A great way to begin is by keeping a folder of clippings for your sigil work. Try the magazine rack or used book rack in a thrift store for interesting materials. Dig through old newspapers.

If you have artistic inclinations, begin making artwork that can be incorporated into your sigils. An image of a bird, for example, can speak to simplicity and freedom, while jewels and pearls can represent abundance. Many images can work for love, like an Irish claddagh, a sacred heart, or a stylized ampersand. Increasing your sense of connection to the universe or to the cosmic unconscious can be facilitated with images that speak of communication: people talking, radio antennae, coiled wires, or coiled serpents.

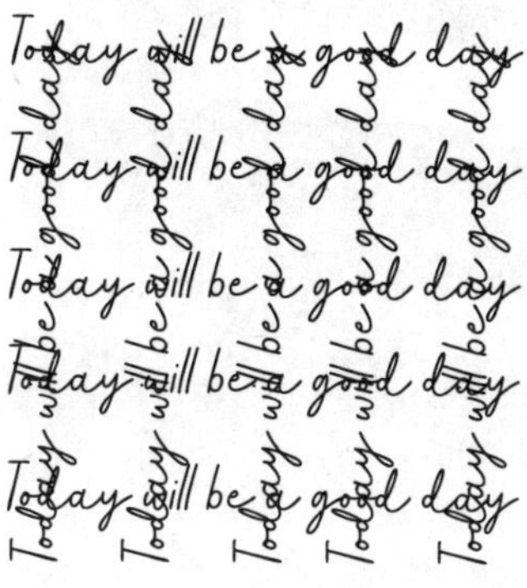

A simple sigil, a magickal square written in cursive in two directions.

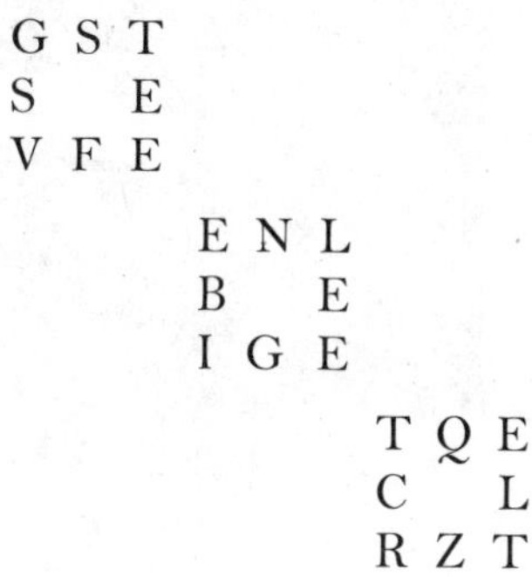

Another sample sigil. You may forget why you initially made a sigil, and that's okay. It will still continue working.

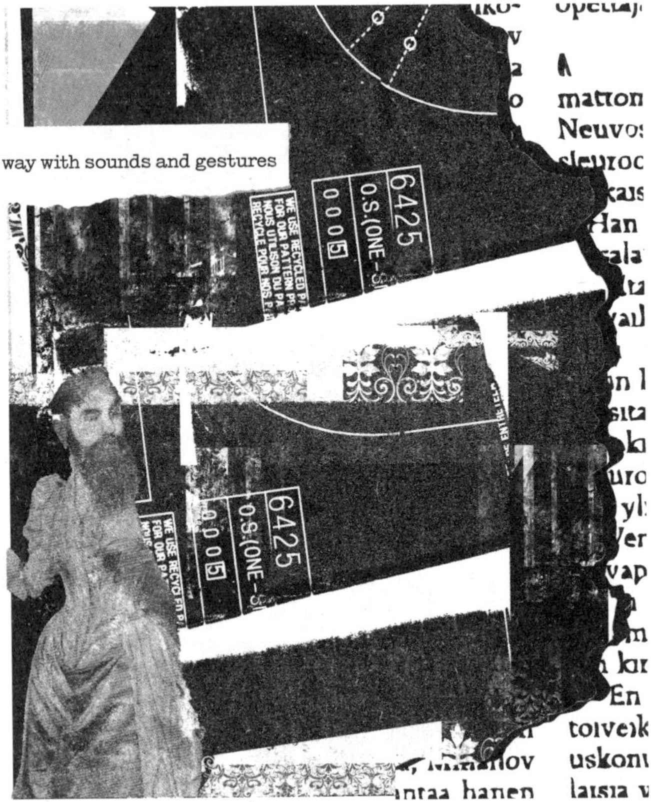

Collage may also be used to good effect.

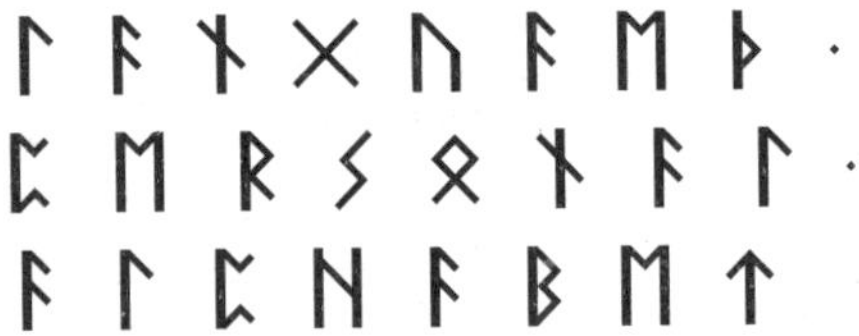

Dead languages and personal alphabets may be employed.

The point is in trying to shake off ordinary perception and take a new point of view. Use your intuition to find materials that speak to you. Acquire photos and texts, even if you don't know precisely how they will be used. Simply take a file folder or a cigar box and fill it with clippings. Add your personal sketches or clip words from old journal entries. As soon as you set the intention of finding materials for your sigil work, the required texts and images will come to you.

Flip the switch. Look at things in a new light. Practice imagining possibility instead of obstacles. Practice awareness instead of slumber. The process described in this chapter requires no astral projection, no consulting the Akashic records, no knowledge of astrology or tarot. And yet the cut-up method can be extremely powerful and results in increased self-knowledge and self-empowerment. The cut-up method helps you to see the difficulties in your life more clearly and move past them through previously unknown means.

Step 2: Creating the Base Text

Often we experience a lack of passion and spontaneity in life because of the power of ingrained habit. We think the same sorts of thoughts, go to the same sort of places, and have the same sorts of conversations over and over again. The heavy weight of habit prevents newness and uniqueness from arising. Magick can help you to scramble ingrained habits and find the exceptional experiences you want. The home of magick lies in interrupting and re-ordering habits of thinking and acting, and the sigil provides a vehicle for this transformation to take place. Through this practice, you will learn to recover a sense of agency in tumultuous times or in situations of everyday tedium.

Begin with what I call the base text. In longhand or on your computer, write a paragraph about the sort of change you want in your life. Try not to censor yourself, and pack a lot of detail into one good paragraph. If you need a word count, think somewhere between one and three hundred words. Don't get too attached to the precise wording, and there is no need to revise and edit. When you are finished, you will have a quick and easy representation of what your conscious mind wants at this point in time. The main thing here is to write freely and quickly so that you don't have a lot of time to second-guess yourself.

If you're having trouble getting started, use a sentence starter. You might try, "It really bothers me when . . ." or "One thing I really want in life is . . ." Or maybe you start with a powerful memory that contains the reality you want to invoke, like a time when you felt especially fulfilled or at peace. Try something like, "I remember the time when . . ." You don't have to be profound or literary or anything like that. Just use your ordinary writing style, like you would write to yourself in a diary or journal. It is perfectly okay if your prose sounds plain, and it is also okay if you want to add your own flourishes.

You can write the base text about anything—it can be a paragraph about something you want to change. Maybe a situation with your boss at work has been bothering you.

Maybe you are trying to attract a new love interest or put together a down payment on a new car. The possibilities are limitless, and you can write about something intensely personal or something affecting the entire planet. Just be honest and direct—no one will read this but you. And, in the next step, you will be cutting and rearranging your base text to get a re-ordered version.

Step 3: Scrambling the Base Text

Now that you have a paragraph about something in your life, you will begin to cut up the paragraph and reassemble it.

One way to do this is to physically print the page and cut it into four quarters. This is the method used by beat writer William S. Burroughs, who wrote, "You cannot will spontaneity, but you can introduce the unpredictable spontaneous factor with a pair of scissors." Reassemble the quarters, so that the first quarter goes with the third and the second with the fourth. You will now have a kind of kaleidoscopic rendering of your paragraph. You can achieve something similar on a computer screen by cutting and pasting the second half of each line into a new location. Finally, you can also cut word-by-word or phrase-by-phrase and reassemble your writing using scissors or a hobby knife and a glue stick.

Now a new paragraph emerges. Much of it will be gobbledygook. It will certainly lack proper grammar in many places, and the punctuation will no longer make sense.

If you like (and this is totally optional), you can add new connecting phrases and punctuation to make the paragraph functional again.

More to the point is to read through the paragraph and look for illuminating or revealing phrases. As you are doing this, you may already begin to find that you see the problem or situation in a new light. Your subconscious or unconscious mind is beginning to speak through the cut-up.

Get a pen or a highlighter and mark the parts that you find to be the most striking or revelatory, the parts that surprised you after you re-assembled your paragraph. As you edit the base text, the temptation will be there to make the new narrative follow a preconceived pathway. Allow the cut-up to breathe its own life, remembering always the risk of making the cut-up say what you think it should say.

Try not to worry too much about readability or form. The key to the crafting of the cut-up or sigil is to allow a message to come through the text that has not been planned in advance, to allow oneself to be interrupted by the process, as though another person were there writing.

Now you can begin to black out or cut away the parts of your paragraph that are extraneous or that do not add anything new. Out of your original paragraph, you will end up with a phrase or a few phrases at the most. These phrases now become the key text, the words that you will use to create your sigil.

Cut these key phrases out of your paper or print them from your computer, since these will be used to create the physical sigil that will be used to work your magickal will. Take these clippings and set them aside while discarding everything else.

Step 4: Creating the Sigil

At this point, you have put a lot of work into the sigil creation process. You collected a file of images from old books and magazines. You wrote the base text, cut it up, and condensed it down into a key text. Now you are ready for the core ritual of the cut-up method of sigil magick. At this point, mindset and setting become more important. You are ready to take the steps of assembling the sigil and charging it.

Begin with the chaosphere meditation or the qabalistic cross exercise. You may want to light some incense and burn a candle or lamp while working. You may also carefully choose a piece of music to play that goes along with the spell.

Once you have performed these preliminaries, set before you the cut-up clippings as well as any images that you plan to use for the sigil. Most importantly, from here forward, concentrate intently upon the result you wish to achieve with this ritual action.

Realize that you, yourself, are not only the agent but also the subject of the change that the ritual will enact. In other words, you must surrender to the ritual action and be willing to change yourself and the way that you do things in order to achieve the desired result. By undertaking this ritual, you are saying to the universe that you are willing and ready to do whatever it takes to ensure the success of the magickal work. Hold this firmness of purpose in mind as you work, yielding your thoughts, feelings, and actions to the ritual at hand.

Open your magickal journal or lay out a separate piece of heavy paper, such as watercolor multimedia paper. Lightly anoint the page with salt water at the four cardinal directions, while saying these words (or similar ones): "I join the work of my hands with my true will. May the sigil I enliven today fulfill its purpose throughout the worlds." The worlds here are all of the many layers of reality, along with the four directions themselves. With these words, you consecrate the ritual space as signifying the entirety of existence.

Now would be the time to invoke any chosen divinities, using the words of the tradition(s) with which you are most familiar. You may also call to mind any departed ancestors or people who have inspired you along the way. Recall also the inner genius or guardian angel, your own higher self. Recall your magickal community, the queer mages who undertake this work along with you. (This step should be kept brief. If you do not know what to say, try something like, "I invite all beneficent spirits present here to aid in this work, to bring it to its successful conclusion.")

Next, paste onto the page the image or images you would like to use. If you are so inclined, add some original artwork of your own. The work should be rapid and intense. Now is not the time to second-guess every line or to perfect your shading technique. Above all, pour your intention into the work, recalling with every slightest movement the purpose for which you are undertaking the ritual.

At this point, you can add your key text to the sigil, the words or phrases that you extracted from your writing. If your phrases are too long to be included, you might use only the initials or only the consonants, eliminating any repetitions. Or the letters might be combined to form a single symbol. Another method is to create a magickal square, writing the phrase in cursive seven times left to right, then rotating the paper ninety degrees and writing it again seven times, directly over what you wrote the first time. The methods are many—the main thing is to get the idea down on paper in some symbolic form. Your text need not be legible, and, for many purposes, it is preferable for it not to be legible.

You now have images overlaid with text. Go with your inner feelings here. If the sigil does not feel complete, keep working. You may add more images or more repetitions of the same text. You may splatter extra paint or ink onto the page. You may feel compelled to cut the paper in a certain way. You may wish to embroider the images with thread or beads. Make sure to recall the purpose for the work at every moment during the ritual. Keep working until you feel that your sigil is complete or until there is simply nothing further that you can do.

The sigil is traditionally charged using bodily fluids. A very simple way to complete this step is to kiss the sigil. This is the way that religious icons are venerated in many traditions. As you do so, say to the now-awakened sigil, "I give you life of my life, breath of my breath, that you may live for the purpose that I have set for you." If you have time, sit for a few minutes in silent contemplation, feeling the energy of the ritual that has transpired. Then simply put the sigil in a safe place and go about your business.

Step 5: After Creating the Sigil

According to some sources, it is better to forget the sigil altogether or even destroy it. I think it is best to retain the sigil and gaze upon it every once in a while to renew the spell. You may place it in a strategic location. Place a love sigil or a dream sigil under your pillow or under the bed. Place a wealth sigil near the center of the home. Place protection sigils near the doorways or windows. Be intuitive about this and do whatever makes sense to you. The right location will have the right feel to it.

Above all, give the sigil time to work. Magick is not a game of slots where you pull the lever and wait for the cherries to align. Magick is about change and transformation. You may see startlingly quick results, or you may sometimes have to wait years to see what you want to occur. Just be patient, and be prepared for the change to come through you. Do not fall into the trap of lust for result: simply see the sigil as an experiment in life that you are conducting.

Allow the sigil to affect your thought processes. Keep in mind that chaos sigils work in nonlinear ways. Pay close attention to your sense of intuition. Guidance may come to you in dreams, or you may find yourself attracted to new places and events. Help may come from an unexpected quarter, like a text from an old friend or a recalled piece of advice. Remain flexible and open.

Step 6: Working with Painful Memories

This book is no substitute for getting professional help from a psychologist or psychiatrist. By all means, use therapy and medications when necessary. But the sigil technique can also help to reframe and transform difficult memories. For LGBTQIA+ people, those memories can often include a coming out or transition experience that did not go well, such as when a friend or relative was not supportive. Some loss is a near universal experience within the LGBTQIA+ community.

You cannot undo the past with the sigil technique, but it may help you to see hidden pathways for growth and understanding that you did not see previously. The sigil technique can also help you to release the hold that painful memories have over you, so that you can begin to heal and move on with your life, with or without the unsupportive person.

To begin, create your sacred space as normal. You may wish to burn a candle and incense, and you will want to do an interior exercise, like the qabalistic cross exercise or the chaosphere meditation.

Then, simply write in longhand about the distressing memory in as much detail as possible. Try to remember with all of your senses what it felt like to be in the room with the person/people who harmed you in some way. Most likely you have already replayed this memory dozens of times—perhaps it already lives on repeat in your head. The difference now is simply that you are getting it down on paper, making it into an external memory, instead of just an internal one.

Try not to censor yourself—it is okay to use profanity if that's what you need to do. You may also experience powerful emotions. You might need to cry or scream a little bit, and that's okay. Just allow those feelings to come and go as they will. Get as much down on the page as you can.

When you come to the end of your account, or if you simply get tired of writing, go ahead and stop. For most people, one to three pages will be enough. It's okay if you don't capture every detail—you can always return to the process later.

Now comes the fun part. By undergoing this process, you are saying to the universe that you are done with this painful memory and the trouble it has caused you. You are saying you are ready for a transformation that will help you see things in a new light and get beyond the hurt.

The physical manifestation of the readiness to move beyond the mental blockage is the cut-up. So, take your scissors or hobby knife and physically cut apart the words of your experience. By doing this, you are not denying that the harmful experience took place or that your feelings are valid. Instead, you are saying that you are ready for change in your life, that you are ready to be rid of the hold that troubling memories have over you. You are submitting your mind and your life to the process of positive transformation. Hold love for yourself in your heart as you do this. Be brave and supportive for yourself. Give yourself all the grace you can.

You should now have in front of you many words and phrases in your own handwriting that you can scramble and reassemble. First, take out the gobbledygook that doesn't make any sense. Then, begin crafting for yourself a new message of your own choosing, a powerful new one that better reflects the way that you want your life to go.

This doesn't have to be like an affirmation or a self-help style mantra. You may just choose to make a silly little poem. Use your creativity and make something of your own. You may extract a new key phrase and make that into a sigil if you like. The important thing to do is to take the negative experience and make it into something positive or at least neutral. You may now decorate your sigil with artwork and keep it some place safe where you can refer back to it, whenever you are feeling powerless or afraid.

Close the experience with some calming music or a few minutes of silence. Try not to rush away from it too quickly. You may notice shifts in your inner outlook right away, but don't try to force anything. You will know the process is working when you feel a sense of calm release. The bad memory will still be there, but you will no longer feel so bound by it. New possibilities will begin to come to mind over the coming days and weeks. You may begin to see yourself or your relationships in a new light.

Step 7: Creating Audio Sigils

You don't really need to use paper and ink to create an effective sigil. Artists like William S. Burroughs and Genesis P-Orridge were known for using audio sampling techniques for magickal practice. For this method, you will only need an audio recording device and, if you want to get fancy with it, editing software like Audacity that has multi-track capacity. For most people, the voice memo app on your phone will do just fine. You could even use old analog equipment like a physical tape recorder if you are feeling low-fi nostalgic. Free sound effects are also available on the internet if you would like to make your sigils more interesting.

Audio sigils work because you can take them with you wherever you go. You can record or play back sigils while on a walk in the park or while driving to work (just be mindful of safety).

For a first take, simply speak your desired outcome into the recording device. This may feel very awkward at first. We often feel uncomfortable speaking our desires out loud, especially for those of us who were raised in very polite or passive-aggressive homes. Speaking desires out loud, even into a tape recorder, is a spell in its own right. Once you have played the recording several times, to the point where you almost have it memorized, you are ready to make a more condensed version.

The condensed version should be a quick phrase, no more than a sentence. Say the phrase, with three repetitions of three. If you feel like dabbling with software, you can loop the phrase nine times or even record it in harmonizing fashion. You can even add a backing track, like meditation music or tanpura. Play the track back to yourself three times a day for seven, thirty, or ninety days.

Pay attention to the effect that background noises have on the magick. Be careful of loud, discordant sounds like ambulance sirens or construction noise that could interfere with the working. You can use such sounds for offensive magick if you are working to disrupt an adversary, but they might not be beneficial for magick based on attraction. Drums and rolling thunder can be used for empowerment, while birdsong and running water can have a calming effect. Don't rule out more technological sounds like FM static or the old dial-up internet sounds, which speak to communication and "dialing in" the right frequency.

Use sounds intuitively in the same way you would use artwork. Each part of your soundscape has a magickal effect. You don't need to control this in an ironclad way though. Chaos itself will aid you in the creation process. Serendipitous sounds will act as part of the "punctuation" of your sigil.

Location also matters when you are playing your sigil back to yourself. If you are looking for creative inspiration, play your sigil in your workspace or studio. If you are looking to attract a lover, play your sigil in your bedroom or right before you walk into a social space, like a party or club. For spells involving money, play the sigil while looking at your finances, like bills or spreadsheets. Playing back your sigil in the appropriate area has the effect of tuning the space to your will, so that the space has a harmonious effect on your psyche.

Don't be obsessive about this though; sometimes you use a space simply because you happen to have some privacy at that space and time. We don't always have the luxury of perfect surroundings, and sometimes even loud backgrounds can feel like home.

Step 8: Remembering the Interior Guide

When creating sigils, make sure to reference your intuition. You will quickly develop an inner guide that will tell you what steps to take, how to begin, and how to conclude the work.

This inner intuition has the greatest significance in magick. Without it, the most ornate ritual will fall flat. With it, a little squiggle on a piece of paper achieves the desired result. Make sure to listen deeply to your inner sense, which will be a constant guide and companion in the magickal arts.

You may sometimes have a hard time accessing this inner sense, and there are no surefire ways to make contact with it. You can increase your chances of accessing intuition by slowing down and not rushing your sigil creation. You might also incorporate some silent meditation into your practice, both before and after your sigil work.

It is also really important to get clear about your true desires before you begin. If you have trouble accessing your intuition, it may be a sign that you have some confusion about what you really want. When this happens, try not to force yourself to a quick conclusion.

If you are feeling uncertain about the direction you want to take in your practice, try writing about your conflicting feelings in your magickal record. Or perhaps do some divination, like a tarot, *I Ching*, or rune reading, to figure out the nature of your own inner life.

Taking long walks outside can also be clarifying, especially when you at least slightly test your physical endurance. Sometimes you just need to get beyond the reach of the conscious mind to find a new approach to a problem.

Additionally, music and artwork can take you to a place beyond the reach of the conscious mind, where intuition begins to open.

Dreams, also, can be a great portal to intuitive understanding, but they may also give you difficult-to-interpret psychic noise. I find the boundary between sleep and waking to be worth exploring. Just before sleep, set an intention of finding clarity in your magickal practice. Ask your spirit guides to show you exactly what is most important at this particular juncture. You may come away with a useful phrase or image for your sigil craft.

Step 9: Clearing Blockages with Sigils

The problem of happiness, and why we fail to find it, boils down to a lack of willingness to change, a blockage in our path. We all want happiness for free, without having to work for it or do anything differently. When it comes to the cut-up, you symbolically submit actions to the process.

The cut-up expresses willingness to change, both at the level of your perception of reality and in the feelings and actions that you project into the world. When you submit writing or audio to the cut-up, the change may come from an unexpected quarter, from some aspect of life considered stable and solid.

Comfort with change seems dangerous and threatening. Part of yourself will crave predictability and certainty. Committing to doing things and thinking in a different way takes courage and strength. Bending toward chaos, complexity, and novelty represents the best way forward from a place of stagnation and dissatisfaction. Your magick takes a leap forward when you commit to fully acting on any guidance that comes your way.

The feeling of being stuck in a rut ends when it is reimagined as only a fleeting appearance. We all create cages of our own devising, in the form of limitations that we place on ourselves. We censor ourselves before we even encounter external resistance. We hobble ourselves with self-doubt and worry. We unconsciously surrender agency on a regular basis. The cut-up supplies a means to push back against the bars of the cage, to find small openings that can be exploited.

After you have completed your sigil, you've opened multiple ways to conquer blockages like the above. You may feel new sensations. Be on the lookout for these small changes and record them in your magickal record.

You may also have smack-you-in-the-face sorts of changes, where you get exactly what you wanted within days of creating the sigil. Just take what comes, whatever that might be. Don't discount the results, whether they are large or small. Commit to taking action when the time comes, and do not shy away from the gifts that chaos brings into your life.

Living into the Work

As you do your sigil work, you will gradually develop your own style of magickal practice. The words and images will flow together smoothly, and you won't second-guess yourself as much. At some point, the ritual becomes not just a quick way to obtain desires but a path to a highly efficient way of life in which every thought focuses on a core purpose.

Ritual points to an entirely different way of living, making inessential things fall by the wayside. With sigils specifically, the ritual becomes word, and when wed with feeling, goes toward the fulfillment of a deeply held interest or goal. The sigil reminds you of what you want to accomplish, in a way that tunes into the senses toward that intent.

This magickal path is a way of avoiding the sort of autopilot approach to life, in which convenience and entertainment matter above all else. Of course, the magickal process can be fun and entertaining, but the primary goal remains the purpose for which you conduct the ritual in question. Along the way, you come to expect surprises and synchronicity, strange forms of assistance, and a plenitude of resources to meet your goals.

At this point in your magickal path, you likely have begun to have some surprises and successes. You may be feeling more comfortable with your LGBTQIA+ identity. You have perhaps experienced more spontaneity and gladness in your life. You have begun to rekindle dreams and desires that you long held dormant. Get excited, because the journey of queer chaos magick continues in the pages ahead.

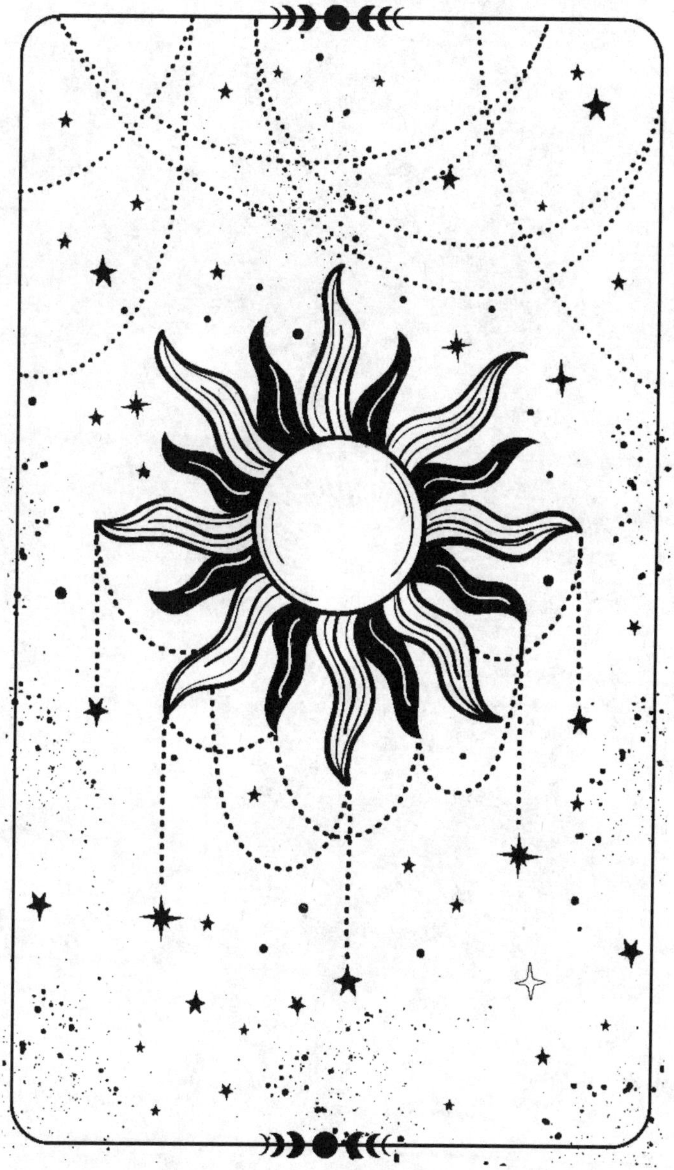

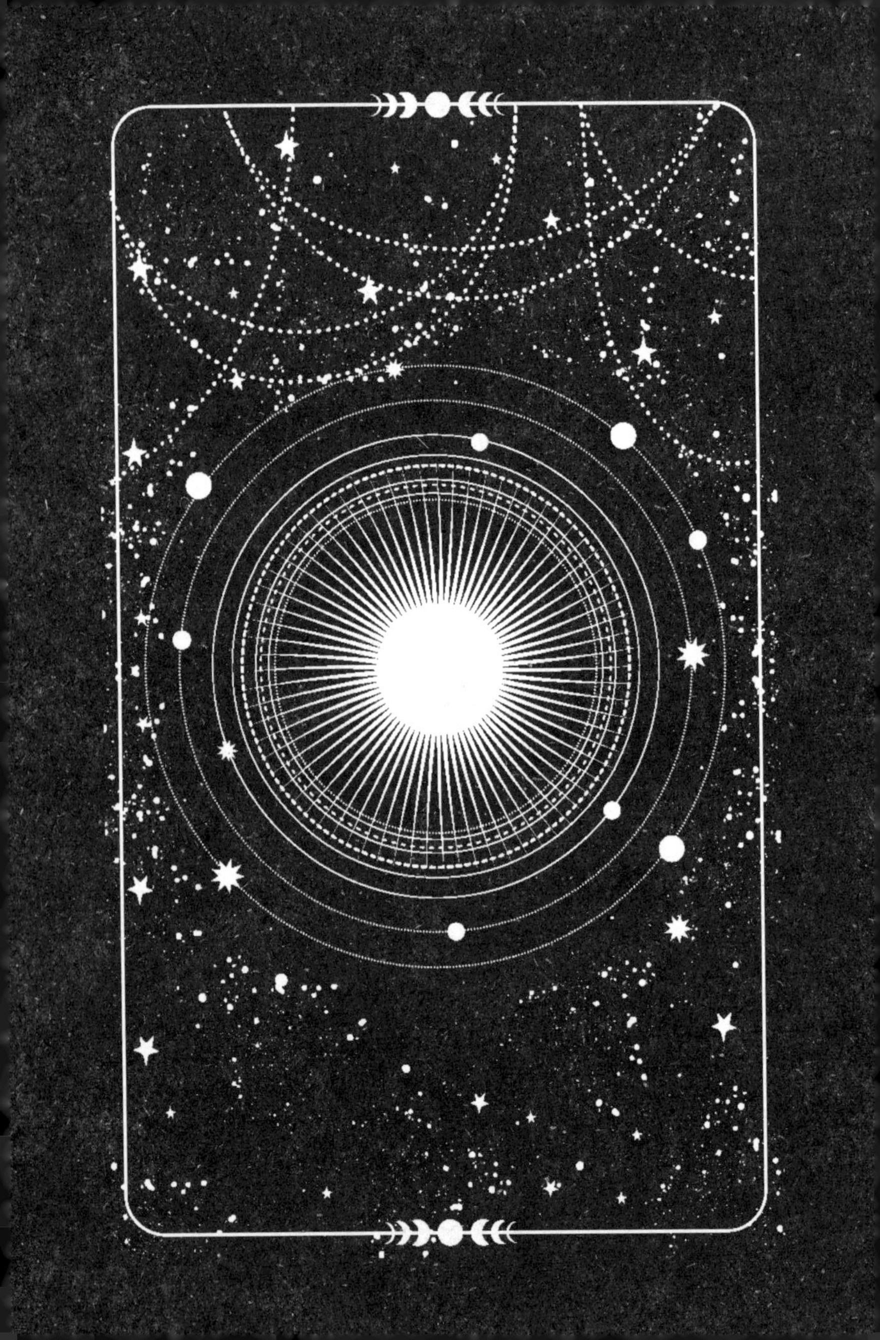

Chapter 4: Chaos Magick and Your Body

In this chapter, through chaos magick, you will explore the human body and gain greater acceptance of your own embodiment, taking into account journeys of transition, of trauma, and of disability. You will go through exercises to appreciate and love your own body so that you get a better sense of your own power. You will get in touch with the "dark light," which helps you to counter homophobia, transphobia, and ableism in society.

Each human body has within it billions of bacterial cells. These microbes help us to digest our food and fight infection. Our bodies are like coral reefs to these bacteria, vast ecosystems in which hundreds of species flourish. We could not live without them, and yet, the idea of bacterial growth seems to us kind of gross. So we use antibacterial soaps and cleaners and overuse antibiotic medications. While some bacteria can be harmful, we cannot purge ourselves entirely of microbes; they are as much a part of us as our human cells. The gut microbiome has been found to interact with our neurology as well, so that the health of the gut has an impact even on our mental health.

The "inside" of our bodies has already been colonized by the "outside" world of microorganisms, so there is no pure point where you begin and the world ends. There are countless ways in which the physical body depends upon the contributions of the world. Your lungs constantly exchange gasses with the atmosphere. The oxygen you breathe was once manufactured by the single-celled organisms in the prehistoric oceans. The light falling on your skin at this very moment comes from a star millions of miles away. Your food ultimately comes from the dirt, which is itself alive and active, an ecosystem in its own right.

To look at the human body, like looking at any ecosystem, is to find complexity within complexity, dependency upon dependency. In a word, chaos.

We should think of chaos not just as mess or disorder, but as intricacy and complexity. And it does not just reside around us, but in our own bodies as well. The body itself is not just a container for our minds, because mind and body are like two sides of the same coin. And our bodies are not just empty containers for the soul. They are important vehicles for self-expression and self-knowledge. Our bodies affect all of our interactions with the world. For this reason, any chaos magician will want to give due attention to the physical body and the psycho-physical exercises that help us to come to terms with it.

Step 1: Honoring Queer Embodiment

Coming out as trans or gay or queer doesn't happen in a vacuum. Transition and coming out happen in the midst of political realities of oppression, division, and hatred, in the face of homophobia and transphobia. We should pay attention to our bodies, because embodiment matters. Bodies matter. Flesh matters. The matter, the materiality of our bodies speaks volumes not only about our own self-expression but also about the kind of world in which we want to live and the hopes we have for the future.

When we open ourselves to being queer, we open that same possibility to others, in the world today and for future generations. This kind of self-revelation and self-disclosure does not happen as a statement of belief only but as self-expression through physical form and intimate relationships as well. Coming out happens through embodiment and through the choices we make with our material selves.

It can be too easy to take embodiment for granted. Each of us has lived in the same body from the day of our birth, and so it comes to seem neutral or invisible to our inner perspectives. At least, when everything goes well, we don't notice our bodies. And yet, the body can never fully be neutral or invisible. This is apparent in discussions about race: white people have the privilege of reading their skin color as neutral and uncomplicated. And in talk of disability, only people who have no health complications or disabilities can have a more or less uncomplicated view of embodiment. And transgender people have not had the experience of seeing their bodies as fully theirs, as straightforward vehicles for self-expression and self-actualization.

Bodies are simultaneously the way that we perceive the world and the way that the world perceives us. They are vehicles for expression, but they are also used by the world to divide and categorize us as people. Bodies can be rendered more or less acceptable depending on how the categorizations fall. We can experience our own bodies as unacceptable through internalized oppression.

Bodies do hold power—to move around through the world, to navigate social spaces, to express style and aesthetics, to bend and twist in interesting ways, to speak and communicate. Bodies also materially link with the built environment and with technology. Through our bodies, we live the rhythms of the world around us. The arm extends to grasp with the hand—the strap on the subway car, the moving handrail of the escalator, or in other embodiments, the grip of the wheelchair or the handle of the cane. We rock with the rhythm of cars and planes, with the beat of the music, with the pulsations of other bodies and other minds. We move our mouths and tongues to the syllables of poetry, to the shock of the latest gossip, to the news and the weather report.

The world courses through the body as music plays through a speaker. The world is experienced through the body, and through the body the world gains expression. This site of physicality is also where the mental world touches the real. The body is both material and ethereal: a bundle of cells and nerve fibers, the recollection of past, and the expectation of the future.

We don't just live in bodies—we live through them and with them. And we also struggle with them, when they don't look or work the way we think they should. Bodies don't behave properly. They resist our intentions for them.

Everyone knows this on some level. Almost everyone has had the feeling of a crick in the neck that just will not go away or not fitting into last year's pants or perhaps breaking a bone and not being able to walk. All bodies fall somewhere on a spectrum of ability and disability. At some point, the fluid motion of the body begins to decompose into pain and dis-ease.

And so it goes with our gendered bodies. Cisgender people, to varying degrees and in shades of difference, experience the body as having an uncomplicated expression that accords with their self-expression. But even here there is discomfort and dysphoria. Cisgender people experience dysphoria in being not muscled enough or in being too muscly, too tall or too short, etc.

Moving further along the gender spectrum, to gender nonconforming and transgender people, the body's expression does not align with the internal vision of selfhood, as though the ideal and the physical have fallen out of sync with one another. The discomfort and dysphoria become strong enough for trans and gender nonconforming people to take steps to better align their ideal, internal version of gender with the gendered expression of the body. And this, of course, is the process of transitioning, which seems simple on paper but is very complicated in all of its legal, social, and medical aspects.

Simply put, honoring the importance of the body is an important part of the invitation to queer chaos magick. Take a moment to meditate on this importance before moving forward.

Step 2: Listening to the Body

As an LGBTQIA+ person, you do not have to accept the jurisdiction of the church, of the courts, or of public opinion over what you do with your body, your love life, the arrangement of your family, or the direction for your future. You have chosen a course in life. You have learned to hear a new music, a new language, through deep listening to your own body, your own story, and your own feelings. You have learned to hear this strange new music, and increasingly, to trust it as leading to freedom.

Poetry and music have an inner resonance and rhythms of their own, just as the body has its own form of knowledge, its own voice. In working with their expressive bodies, transgender and gender nonconforming people accept the materiality that they have been given to create new forms, new metaphorical music. These new forms are in continuity with the old but also bring about ruptures and breakages with the past.

In learning to listen to your own body and desires, you necessarily decouple from the paths in life previously charted for you by your family background and any other tribes to which you belong.

For transgender and gender nonconforming people, this kind of detachment occasions both bliss and exhaustion. A great relief comes from no longer having to perform the gender assigned at birth or the sexual mores of the larger society. And yet the feelings of euphoria also come with great pain and loss. Pain at the loss of time before you released yourself from the illusions of society, pain at being misunderstood, pain at being labeled as dishonest or deceptive or having your feelings minimized or explained away.

By coming out, LGBTQIA+ people launch into a much more uncertain and precarious future, marked by economic difficulties, transphobic and homophobic harassment, loss of at least some of our relationships, and for some at least—for black trans women in particular—the real danger of physical violence. Euphoria goes hand in hand with exhaustion as you navigate your way through a world that has not been built with queer or especially transgender people in mind, that makes you bend over backwards to get name changes, hormone treatments, and surgeries or to have the sort of marriage and family you want.

There is a real solidarity here with people with disabilities navigating a world that views some bodies as normal and others as aberrant, some bodies as worthy and others as freakish. The built environment itself separates us into forced binaries of male and female, able and disabled, as though these markers of identity were simple on/off switches. But of course, you do not fit neatly into masculine or feminine, able or disabled categories. You find yourself born queer or born transgender, just as you might be born with mental or physical illness or develop disabilities later in life.

Since you cannot "pray away the gay" or will away your own peculiar embodiment, you take that which society labels as a defect and make it into power. You no longer want to be normal and acceptable. You no longer want to play it safe by trying to hold to the norms you inherited. You accept your queer embodiment, your body with disabilities, your own strange self that has been through so much history with so many scars. You seek to give yourself, your body, and your mind the care that you missed along the way.

You need not wait for a perfected body, an absolved body, a conquered body in order to love your own embodiment. You begin with a love for your own imperfections, your own queer body, your "broken" body, your painful body, and accept it as it is, while at the same time acknowledging the place for adornment and modification, expression and eroticism.

Your body is being and becoming at the same time, a plastic site of expansion and contraction, situated halfway between the real and the desired, the desired and the desirable. The opposite of terror and hatred is self-love and self-forgiveness, the refusal to go on hating your physical self, to give yourself the expression denied for so long.

In light of all of this, take a few moments to listen to your body before proceeding to the next steps.

Step 3: Writing a Love Letter to the Body

Open your sacred space with a few minutes of silent meditation, taking the time to notice your physical form and how it feels at this moment in time. You may notice random aches and pains—some lower back trouble, perhaps, or a stiff neck or a headache. Breathe into these problem areas and give your body loving attention. You may begin to feel the surface of your skin as it meets the air around you. You may feel your breath as it rises and falls. You may notice the space between your eyes. The interior of your body may come to seem like a vast, cavernous space. Take a few minutes to dwell in the inner space while also noticing your physical form, as well as any sensations that come to you.

At this point, allow yourself to do something that may feel awkward, weird, and difficult. Open your magickal record and write a love letter to your physical body. Address your body as beloved or some other honored designation. Try to speak to it in a kind and warm way, like you are speaking to an old friend. Here are some of the prompts that you can use to write your letter:

Let me tell you some of the things that I love about you . . .

I see how much you struggle to . . .

I appreciate the way that you . . .

In the future, I want for you . . .

I will take care of you by . . .

As you write, notice that you have a relationship with your own body, just like you might have with another person. Cultivate inside a love for your body.

You may notice feelings of resistance coming to the fore from time to time. You may have deep-seated feelings of hatred for the body. You may have a past history of self-harm, substance abuse, or an eating disorder that has left you scarred in some way. You can acknowledge the existence of these old feelings without letting them control you. Just keep insisting on holding your body in love and acceptance.

Keep repeating to yourself phrases like, "I love you. I am thankful for you. I will take care of you." After a few minutes, write some good things you can do to take care of yourself and love your physical form.

Note that you may need to repeat this exercise from time to time. You may have old feelings of self-loathing come creeping back. You may look in the mirror and not like what you see. Just keep going back to the exercise. After many repetitions, you will begin to feel more at home in your own skin and more able to deal with dysphoria and any troubling emotions that arise.

Step 4: Recognizing the Body in Process

Your body is at once yours, and, at the same time, you never quite control it. Your body has its own priorities that resist attempts to strictly govern it. Your body has its own story, rooted in the past, unfolding in the present, and arcing toward the future. The body can be felt in these three modes, as an artifact of things accomplished, as an expression of current life, and as a vehicle for not-yet-present realities. This long arc of desire manifests itself in the physical form, which receives impressions from the world. To work with the body in a way that does not cause harm, we have to understand it in a loving way, to learn to read its story and hear its song.

Begin by bathing and changing into very comfortable clothes. Center yourself using the chaosphere meditation. Light a lamp that symbolizes love. This might be a pink salt lamp or a rose-colored candle. You might place a piece of rose quartz in your meditation space. Play some soft music without any lyrics, something you find calming and peaceful. Burn soft incense like rose or cedar, but avoid overdoing it. Finally, consecrate a large piece of paper or some blank pages in your magickal record with a smudge of ash or some sprinkles of water.

Divide your paper or pages into three segments. Mark the three segments as "past," "present," and "future."

Begin by writing about your body's history, in full paragraphs if you like, or you may use bullet points or notes. The past of your body should include any scars you have, any broken bones or places of pain, or any other remnants of past trauma. Map onto the body your memories of past events. As you do so, hold in your heart the intention for healing, wholeness, and wellness.

Now, turn your attention to the way your body feels in this present moment. Note any places of pain or tension as well as any sensations you might be feeling. Perhaps you are aware of the contact of the air on your skin or the drape of your clothing. Perhaps you notice your belly or your chest rise and fall with your breathing.

Take the time to appreciate your body for the features that you love. Forgive your body, as well, for the ways it does not live up to the standards you set for it. Set the intention to heal and release any harsh judgements you may have about your physical form or appearance. Write all of these thoughts down in your magickal record or on a separate piece of paper.

Finally, write your desired future for your body, willing for this vision to come true as you write. Perhaps think of any transition-related changes you would like to make, like going on hormone replacement therapy or having top or bottom surgery. Or maybe think of your ideal fashions and adornments. Perhaps think of any physical exercise or healthful diet you would like to give your body. Avoid shaming here entirely, and do not conjure any visions of harsh discipline of the body (unless that's your thing).

This is just your chance to fantasize about your body and what you would like to do with it in the future. Take a moment to dwell here in this vision as you write, as though everything you can imagine will come true. Take the time to really fan the flames of belief and craft a good image of your embodiment for the future.

When you have finished, take your bodily vision and seal it in some way, perhaps with a wax seal, a monogram, or a signature. Keep your vision in a safe place, and return to it whenever you are feeling like you need a boost in your body image or you are looking for inspiration. Above all, look upon your physical form with love, and invoke all of the blessings that you can. Remember the past, present, and future of your body, and take time every day to cherish it as much as you can.

Step 5: Banishing Shame through the Luminous Darkness

The "dark light" or "luminous darkness" is a real phenomenon that can be found through meditation and introspection. To get in touch with it, sit in silence while looking within. Close your eyes, and breathe deeply. You will begin to experience the interior space, particularly the head and the chest cavity, as a kind of inner cave or hollow.

At first, it will seem completely blank and void. Then, you will find that you can conjure nearly any object via the inner senses through the faculty of imagination. Finally, by detaching from the imagination, you can simply sit still while attending to the inner darkness, void, or emptiness. The attention will tend to wander. Simply bring your mind back to this inner space and observe.

As you breathe in and out, picture a current of energy moving from the base of your spine up to the crown of your head and out. The energy then cycles around your body, forming a large ovoid sphere that extends out from your body several feet in any direction.

With each inhalation and exhalation, the current flows up your spine and out the crown of your head. You may begin to see flecks of color pass before your mind's eye, or you may begin to see rays of light moving upwards. If you don't have this experience, do not worry. Simply sit in silence and observe the interior space. You don't need to be rigid with this practice: try it for five, ten, fifteen, or twenty minutes. If you have time and inclination, see if you can move up to an hour.

The next part is crucial. You don't need to be in formal, seated meditation to experience the dark light, or what may be called a state of interior bliss. You can experience it any time you simply attend to your embodiment and take pleasure from nothing other than simple consciousness, simply being alive and aware.

Think about the feeling of being warm and in your bed, surrounded by the coziness of your pillows and blankets. Or consider the feeling of sitting in your favorite chair, drinking a cup of coffee or tea. Or think about the feeling of a break at work, when you have a few minutes with nothing to do. The point here is that quietness and solitude can be enjoyable in its own right. Sometimes, within this state of quiet rest, a feeling of boundlessness will arise within, as though your own body contains infinity. This is the luminous darkness that can be cultivated and strengthened for the purpose of magickal work.

Now that you have learned to cultivate the dark light, you may use it to banish negative experiences and feelings from the past. When you are in your safe ritual space, take a few minutes to reflect on the ways you may have been shamed in the past because of your sexual orientation or gender identity.

Maybe someone made you feel ashamed because you wore clothes deemed inappropriate for your gender assigned at birth.

You may have experienced subtle or overt bullying because you dressed too masculine or too feminine.

Or maybe you liked toys or games you were not "supposed" to like.

Or maybe you liked TV shows or movies that did not fit with your assigned gender role.

Take a minute or two to feel the hurt and shame of those times, and then, firmly and from the core of your being, say to yourself, "I banish shame through the power of the luminous darkness." Repeat a second and a third time if necessary.

Next, turn your attention to your embodiment, to those places in your relationship with your own body that still give you discomfort.

Maybe you have been shamed because of the shape of your body. Maybe you were made to feel ashamed because your body has been labeled as too fat or too thin, too soft or too muscly.

Maybe you have been shamed for not being athletic enough or for being too athletic.

Or it could be features that have been targets for bullying and microaggression, perhaps because of your racial background or skin tone.

Or perhaps you have facial features that have made you feel ashamed. Perhaps you have been teased or felt dysphoria about the shape of your nose or chin, or your hairline or jawline.

Or maybe you feel awkward or ashamed of your relationship with clothing and adornment, like your clothes never fit appropriately or look the way you want them to look. Maybe this has been a source of distress for you.

Bearing all these things in mind, firmly and from the center of your being, say to yourself, "I banish shame through the power of the luminous darkness." Repeat a second and a third time if necessary.

Finally, consider your relationship with ability and disability. Perhaps you were made to feel ashamed because of factors beyond your control, like the way you carry your body.

Perhaps you were shamed for using assistive technology, like glasses, a cane, a wheelchair, or a hearing aid.

Perhaps you were made ashamed because of your mode of communication, such as through signing or typing.

Think now of all of the ways in which you were made to feel that your body is wrong in some way, for no other reason than your difference as compared with others.

Perhaps you were made ashamed because of a medical condition or mental illness that you have, or because of your regimen of medications and therapies.

Perhaps you were made to feel ashamed because of your need for accommodations at work or school or because you couldn't adequately feign a standard of "normality" as compared to your peers.

Perhaps you have experienced subtle or overt discrimination in your work or personal life because of your disability.

Bearing these things in mind, firmly and from the center of your being, say to yourself, "I banish shame through the power of the luminous darkness." Repeat a second and a third time if necessary.

After performing these banishings, take a few minutes to sit quietly in the interior calm. You may feel a sense of lightness or relief overtake you, as well as a sense of courage and empowerment.

Take the time to revel in your difference from other people. Experience and own that difference or uniqueness. Feel your difference, your weirdness, your queerness, as part of what makes you strong and capable. And if you do not feel a sense of empowerment or relief, that's okay as well. It is okay to feel overwhelmed by your life circumstances, to feel as though you would rather just be that illusory "normal" sometimes.

Let the dark interior light be a source of comfort and shelter for you in difficult times. Take a minute or two to give thanks for whatever you experience in this moment. Close with some words that occur to you, or say the following: "I take the luminous darkness as my solace and strength. I do not shoulder my burdens alone, but by the strange light within me, I find my path and my kin. I give thanks for this darkness inside myself, which I take as my guide and wellspring."

Step 6: Dismantling Christofascism

In the world today, especially in the United States, the Christian right is on the march, with hundreds of laws taking aim at abortion rights and transition care and even seeking to ban LGBTQIA+ books and drag shows. In this time, we take refuge in the dark light within ourselves, within the queer community, and within the praxis that we set for ourselves, in public demonstrations and acts of resistance.

One of the major symbols of rebellion against the authority of the church and theocracy in general, is, of course, the devil, Lucifer, or Satan. Lucifer is a bringer of light, the luminous darkness you learned to cultivate in the above exercise. In contrast to a light that comes from above, Luciferean light comes from within, in the divine knowledge held within the darkness of our own hearts. In contrast to the need for external authority figures and revealed texts, chaos magick disrupts the hierarchical, patriarchal logic of domination. In contrast to the singular Truth of the church, chaos magick rejects enforced dogmas and seeks multiple paths to truth.

Now that you have completed the meditations in this chapter, you may wish to put in your home shrine or meditation space a black candle or an image of Lucifer to represent the dark light of Satanic illumination. Take the time to cultivate the dark light when you engage in sacramental acts of resistance, such as seeking abortion care, taking hormone replacement therapy, or planning for artistic or political resistance.

In contrast to the light of traditional religion, you will not feel the same need to abase or negate yourself in order to seek solace. You need not set aside your intellect, your willfulness, or your sense of humor in order to engage with the Prince of Darkness, who meets you exactly as you are at the crossroads within the chaosphere. Satan or Baphomet acts as the ultimate filter for all kinds of religious hypocrisy. When you embrace Satanic symbolism, false piety falls away from you, and you learn to embrace your true self as well as the creativity and camaraderie of Satanic community.

Most of the people reading this book will have some kind of religiously-based trauma as a result of having been rejected or shamed because of the bigotry of the Christian community in particular. Nevertheless, you may feel a sense of loss at the relationships you left behind or the time invested in trying to fit into a monotheistic worldview.

You may now begin to realize that you are dealing with a sunk cost fallacy, that you are mourning for time lost that cannot be reclaimed, and that leaving the Church later in life is better than never having left at all. Many of the friendships that you may have had in the church were actually very weak. Indeed as very few people, if any, were willing to come with you on your journey into queerness or transness. Even many liberal-minded churchgoers remain infected with a kind of addiction to a certain image of decency that precludes affiliation with the outcasts from the church. The loss of the old community of the church is now replaced with the fellowship of those who uphold the luminous darkness of chaos.

In place of the closed community of the church, you now embrace a loose style of affiliation, the community of those who have chosen the path of chaos. Every time you share something of chaos magick with like-minded others, you strengthen the ties of queer community and thwart the cisheteropatriarchy. Going to the inner well of the dark light enables you to keep going even when it seems that the deck is stacked against you.

The community of like-minded practitioners will keep you going even in the face of homophobic and transphobic bigotry. Seek sincerely the community of queer chaos magick, and it will appear to you. Allow the dark light to guide you into the hidden fellowship of others who share the same vision for bodily autonomy and queer joy.

Step 7: Cursing the Cishetero-ableist Patriarchy

It is not unethical to cast curses in self-defense or to protect vulnerable communities. Curses can be cathartic for the practitioner, allowing some sense of respite from the harm caused by an abuser. Curses can also set into motion an unseen chain of events that brings about greater justice and equity. When we curse someone in a deserving sense, we take their own negative energies and bring them to bear on their own heads. We do not will harm; we simply ask that the law of karma work in an expedited fashion.

You can use this procedure for anyone or anything. Just use it sparingly: this is not the kind of thing you want to do for the annoying person in front of you at the checkout line. Save it for the big stuff.

Below you will find a generalized ritual for the enemies of the queer community.

The materials you will need are a plate, salt, a vessel of water, a cloth, some paper, and a pen. You may also choose a musical playlist that feels aggressive and/or empowering. (Think "Eye of the Tiger" meets "Satan Worshipping Doom.")

Say: *By the salt of the primordial oceans, I purify this plate, this time, this place. May this salt burn in the wounds of my enemies. May the oppressor never find succor, rest, or peace. May the cruel tyrant burn with unquenchable thirst. May the legions of hypocrites in the church be exposed, cast out, and destroyed.* Sprinkle salt on the plate. *As the slug writhes in salt, so does my enemy.*

Say: *With this water, I purify this place as well as my own mind and heart. I understand with great clarity, within and without, my place within the great flux of things.* Sprinkle the water in the four directions and then touch it to your forehead, your breast, and your stomach. *May this inundation undermine, dilute, and fragment the opposition in the halls of power.* Pour the water on the salt and watch it dissolve. *May the unjust politicians lose everything and their plans come to nought.*

Say: *I write here with paper and quill the names of those who have harmed me and those I love. I write these names upon the fabric of the universe, and I ask that those so named be destroyed or otherwise separated from the community.* Write the names in plain text, in cipher, or in an unknown or dead tongue. Place the piece of paper in the water on the plate. *May those who have harmed us be reduced to nothing. May they be erased and forgotten. May all who gained unjustly be brought to account.*

Say: *May those who, with hatred and ignorance, harm the immigrant community, harm people of color, harm the sick and disabled, and harm the LGBTQIA+ community be utterly stamped out, reviled, brought low, and ripped asunder. May those who curtail the rights of women and those who harm children be utterly stamped out, reviled, brought low, and ripped asunder. May this be done in the light of day so that all may see. So mote it be.*

Cover the plate with the cloth and leave it in the same place until the next day. If anything remains of the paper, burn it in an unconsecrated fire. Pour the water that remains in a deserted place. If possible, shatter the plate and throw the shards in the trash. Use the cloth for cleaning the bathroom. When all of the remains of the ritual have been cleared, place a flower arrangement or something soothing, such as a candle or a bell, in the place where the work took place.

Embodiment and the Road Ahead

In this chapter, you took a close look at your relationship with your physical form. You worked on repairing old wounds and established a loving relationship with yourself. You made some plans for how you want to treat your body in the future. Along the way, you discovered the luminous darkness in the cave of your own heart, and you learned to trust that darkness as a source of refuge and strength.

The path of chaos magick does not go in a straight line. It loops and twists back on itself. So, in the months to come, you may experience old habits coming back again. You may sometimes find yourself criticizing your body in the mirror or getting back into destructive habits. At that point, you may want to repeat the rituals in this chapter. The journey of self-love can be long and difficult, but know that you have already made significant progress.

You have learned to love yourself as a queer person. You have learned to stop hiding who you are from the world. You are living into your uniqueness and becoming your full self. You are attuning yourself to the chaos at the heart of the universe, and the chthonic forces support you in your journey to healing and wholeness. The forces of bigotry and ignorance cannot stop you from becoming your full self.

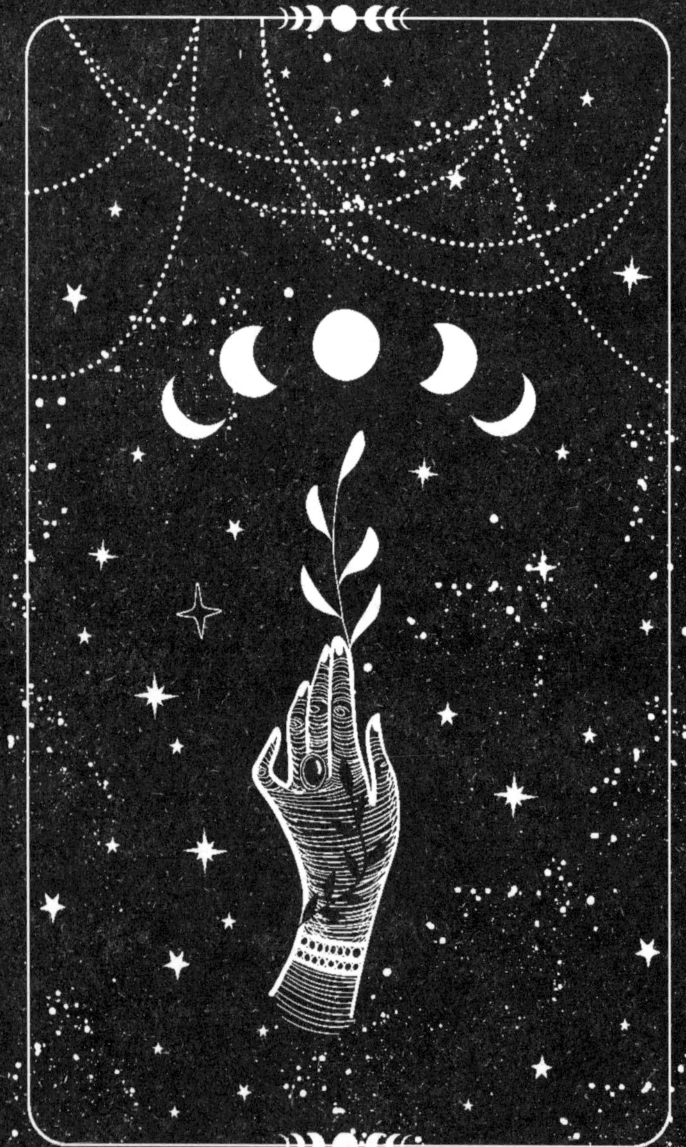

Chapter 5: Finding Your True (Queer) Will

By embracing chaos and through some simple divinations, you can discover your true will—your life's purpose. By the end of this chapter, you will have great insight into your true aim, and you will have confidence that will help you to take action.

We face challenges in our lives not just because of the outward forces acting against us, but because of the internalized powerlessness we learn from society. Magick is the process of uncovering what we really want and then projecting that outwards into reality. Magick is a process of both discovery and empowerment.

Queer, transgender, and gender nonconforming people come out of the closet in order to live in accordance with their true will or deeper self. Occultist Aleister Crowley defined true will as that which lies beyond societal conventions: "Do what thou wilt shall be the whole of the law," and yet willing goes beyond what one feels like doing at any given moment. Living according to true will means living according to your highest artistic, spiritual, and philosophical aims, living according to the dictates of your inner self.

Living according to your true will often means shedding the expectations of tradition, stepping outside of a conventional belief system and into something exceptional and different. At the same time, true will does not require setting aside your temporal, fleshly self but instead is about harnessing the body's power for the possibilities of infinite self-expression. True will is not mere hedonism but a purposeful, transformative route to draw the appetites into the search for inner meaning.

You may not always know when you are acting in accordance with true ill or not, since the path of chaos magick is dark and difficult and there is a tension between your higher self and the part of you that has been wounded by the world. In the process of chaos magick, you are gradually learning to integrate your motives, drives, and desires into a path filled with purpose and meaning.

To find and express true will, you must get more comfortable with pushing the boundaries of acceptability, to live more fully into queerness and difference. The danger usually lies in playing things safe, in wanting to conform with social expectations, in seeking career and material advancement. Queerness must maintain its association with alternative expressions of sexuality, but it should also mean being weird, strange, and different.

Your queer will takes chances on artistic expression and personal freedom. It seeks uncommon and subversive experiences. It bends and breaks systems of oppression. It goes into uncomfortable places and challenges the status quo. But at the same time, your damaged self, ravaged by the forces of control, seeks comfort, safety, and stability.

This sets up a basic tension inside yourself, between the higher self that wants to explore and the wounded child that wants to remain safe. The goal of the practice of queer chaos magick is to create space for experimentation while still feeling supported and loved.

Through it all, remember that queerness supports itself, in that community finds community. You create community in the form of supportive voices: voicing support for yourself, editing the internal critic, and cultivating a supportive spirit.

Together then, let us go on a journey to find your true (queer) will.

Step 1: Magick and the Control Society

In the 80s and 90s, artist Genesis P-Orridge and other collaborators revived Crowleyan magick in a new, more fluid and contemporary form in Thee Temple ov Psychick Youth (TOPY). The group brought mixed media, such as collage, audio, and video, into the construction of sigils while retaining Crowley's emphasis on true will and the transformative potential of sex. The TOPY network led to the formation of many musical projects, including the bands Psychic TV and Throbbing Gristle, credited with founding industrial music and contributing to rave culture.

Early practitioners of body modification and the BDSM scene were also among those aligned with the TOPY ethos and social network. The term *occulture* originated with P-Orridge and captured the sense that the purpose of magick was not just inward-looking ceremonies but the transformation of culture itself.

Another sense of occulture arises from the TOPY writings: any form of expression can potentially become ritual. And rituals have the aim of uniting the conscious and unconscious selves, leading the practitioner into a higher quality, more individualized way of life.

The antithesis of magick is what the TOPY writings call control, a kind of psychic flattening produced by mass society, characterized by mindless conformity and mediocrity, following along with the dictates of the state, the church, the family, and other institutions of technological, capitalist society. The practice of magick opens the door to seeing new possibilities, new realities, precluded by prevailing modes of thought. The TOPY techniques seek to shock participants into seeing the effects of control and finding ways around its deadening grip.

TOPY no longer exists in an organized form, but queer magickal or spiritual practitioners today can learn from the "psychick" teachings and use them in the journey of queerness, creating a neo-TOPY that makes queerness into a spiritual and artistic process. In other words, neo-TOPY is the opening of new terrains, new places and possibilities, through the use of queer occult practices.

The forces of control—especially right-wing political and religious figures—want to make the journey of queerness, and especially of transition, seem like a dead end, so that genderqueer people encounter only obstacles. The viciousness of patriarchal society, its utter indifference for human well-being, can be felt in employment and housing discrimination and through online and real-life harassment. A host of laws in the U.S. and Europe also seek to curtail access to gender-affirming care and make existing in public as a queer person illegal.

But here, our purpose is not to detail the queerphobic efforts of control, but instead to see through and work around them by using occulture. The work of queer magick today lies in finding doors instead of walls, lines of flight through which self-expression can utterly conquer and crush bigotry and exclusion.

This happens not through forgiveness of the oppressor or through some form of universal love, but rather through unapologetic fidelity to a queer, liberatory artistic vision. This vision unfolds through writing, artwork, and ritual, shared among a community of like-minded individuals who seek together to overcome the forces of control and create spaces for creativity and difference. The path to transformation and liberation cannot be found through a ready-made doctrine or method, but the queer chaos philosophy provides some starting points for queer liberation today.

The unconscious or sleeping person, who lives according to control, predetermines the limitations they are willing to accept, in effect dooming artistic endeavors before they begin. In other words, a blocked artist assumes that most things are not possible, which then becomes an excuse for a lack of exertion.

By contrast, the aware person still has hard limits that must be faced, but they are not predetermined at the outset. This artist will plunge headlong in the effort, not knowing exactly where the limits or boundaries are.

Simply put, the person in the control mindset believes that they understand the world and their predetermined place in it, while the magickal practitioner views the world as an unfolding mystery that can be shaped through a process of artistic and occult engagement. Understanding these truths is an important first step in finding your true will.

Step 2: Invoking Chaos

Magick and art express the same impulse of stepping outside of the usual and into the realm of the surprising, the uncanny, and the mystifying.

Try this exercise to liberate routine from boredom and complacency. Begin at your workspace, whether that be an office, a classroom, a cubicle, a store, or a factory. Find a surface that no one will see right away, like the underside of a counter

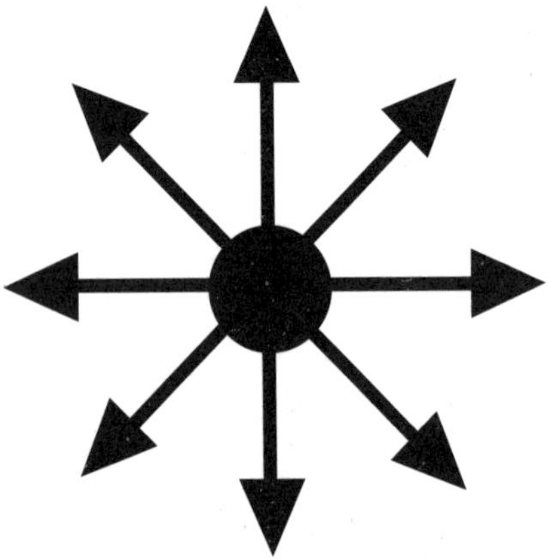

A symbol of chaos magick, with arrows radiating in eight directions.

or the bottom of a laptop, and trace there a symbol of chaos magick. This might be a circle with arrows radiating in all directions or a sigil of your own design. If you are in a place that will allow it, burn a black candle and some clarifying incense, such as cedar or copal.

As you trace the symbol, say something like the following: "I invite the disruptive forces of chaos into this place. I look for the torrent of change in the midst of the same. I unbind myself from drab routines, and I embrace the newness that comes to me today. I will notice uniqueness as it passes my eye, and I devote myself to the second sight." Whenever you get a free moment throughout the day, take a minute to reaffirm these words and touch your magickal symbol again with your fingertip.

After you have placed your symbol and said the charging words, your work begins. Look for anything out of the ordinary that catches your eye. You might see a person wearing a bright red scarf, or a stranger may come into your life. You might receive a business opportunity. You may see changes in the weather or unexpected events in the news. Give silent thanks to chaos for bringing even the slightest bit of newness and change into your life. Watch also your reactions to change as it comes. Just be on the lookout for anything weird, and note also your inner states of mind.

Within yourself, you sometimes may notice a curmudgeonly attitude toward change, a kind of instinctive negative reaction to anything different. You will want to work with this attitude and try to find the positive side of change, even for events that seem to work against you.

Nothing can happen to you that does not hold sweetness as well as bitterness, risk as well as reward.

Watch also your inner senses. You may begin to have intuitions about the motivations of people who come into your life—not necessarily reading their thoughts, but having insight into their true desires. You may also receive little hints about how to approach your work so that it becomes more invigorating and satisfying.

Step 3: Short-Circuiting Control with the Planets

By taking a close look at your life, you may feel very stuck in some parts, while you feel more free in others. Maybe your love life is going well, but your rent is too high and you have a mountain of bills to pay. Or maybe your finances are in good shape, but your job feels exceedingly dull or stressful.

Of course, every life has its ups and downs, problems and difficulties, but you naturally want to get to a point where nothing feels terribly wrong or overwhelming. Your magickal practice should have one aspect that helps you see through self-imposed limitations and another that helps you break through outside barriers.

Sometimes it can also feel overwhelming to tackle all aspects of life at once, so you want to know where to concentrate your efforts for maximal results. To short-circuit control in your life, it can help to have a quick method of divination to use on-the-go, so that you can understand a problem in short order, perhaps when you do not even have tarot cards or an astrology chart handy. Instead of the standard twelve houses of astrology, use the below abbreviated system of nine houses, with the following meanings ascribed to them:

1. The soul, the self, the internal landscape
2. Money, material resources, business partnerships
3. Research, study, writing
4. Home, the hearth, family
5. The soul, creativity, romance
6. Physical health, work-life balance, self-care
7. Life partnership, commitment, soul mates
8. Religion, philosophy, the occult
9. Journeys, exploration, insight

Number a tic-tac-toe board one through nine, randomly or in sequential order, corresponding to the above nine houses.

Now make nine paper tokens or number nine coins, corresponding to the nine astrological planets/celestial bodies, listed below with quick associations:

1. The Sun: revelation, blessings, leadership
2. The Moon: devotion, receptivity, transformation
3. Mercury: communication, speech, understanding
4. Venus: luxury, beauty, abundance
5. Mars: strife, aggression, effort
6. Jupiter: wisdom, insight, harmony
7. Saturn: stagnation, lethargy, harshness

8. Rahu (the north node of the moon): expansion, ascension, activation
9. Ketu (the south node of the moon): contraction, descension, compression

Use a random number generator, such as Random.org, to associate the planets with houses, keeping in mind that sometimes more than one planet may occupy the same house. For example, the number pair, 8-1 could mean Rahu in the first house. Keep going until all planets have been assigned to houses. Place coins or tokens on the tic-tac-toe board so that you have a visual representation of the position of the planets. By the time you have finished assigning your planets to houses, you should have a complete picture of your life, a snapshot of where everything stands at that particular moment in time.

Notice that we are severing all pretense of a connection between astronomy and astrology. Notice also that we have simplified the usual twelve houses down to just nine, largely for convenience and compactness. We are simply using the planets as symbols for the inner workings of the subconscious mind, much as might be done with the inkblots of a Rorschach test.

Look for places of strength in particular. Mercury in the third house might be particularly beneficial for writing a book or studying a new topic. Venus in the fifth house might portend romantic attraction. Here, you are creating not so much a complete astrological chart as a thumbnail sketch of what is happening in your life at the present moment.

A simple way to read your mini-chart is in terms of strengths and weaknesses. Look for the places in your life where you have an opportunity to grow. You may be able to study a new subject, add connections to your network, or learn a new skill. Set yourself a few simple goals for these areas of strength.

Take the time also to pay attention to your weaknesses. Oftentimes, Saturn will signal an area of weakness, as it is a slow-moving, cold planet. You might also take cues from the contracting energies of Ketu, the south node of the moon, as indicating areas where energy is waning. If you have Saturn or Ketu in an area of your chart, it does not necessarily spell doom. It may just be that now is a time for rest and regrouping.

This method allows you to look at your life outside the forces of control, centering instead the forces of chaos.

Step 4: Transgressing Boundaries and Dealing with Guilt

As an LGBTQIA+ occult practitioner, you already have some experience with breaking the societal molds. You have probably had a good deal of gender-bending in your life, and your romantic partners have set you apart from straight society. This experience on the margins has given you a great deal of camaraderie with artists and mystics, revolutionaries and reformers.

Your journey from here is one of continuing to break molds and shatter expectations, one of living life on your own terms, not on the ones dictated to you by society. You can step into your magickal strength by holding on to your ability to transgress boundaries.

We may come to magick for very specific reasons, such as a desire for money, sex, or power. But we stay because we find our entire worldview has changed, to one of open exploration of the weirdness—the queerness—that operates at the heart of reality.

In order to continue on this journey of exploration, we have to identify the areas where we still feel stuck and then make steps towards transgressing the boundaries we have inherited.

For those raised in very religious homes, transgressing boundaries may involve working on an acceptance of sexuality and any other form of abundance or luxury in life. In those cases, it can be beneficial to work with magick a bit outside of your comfort zone, that feels a bit out of reach.

For those with challenges accepting the sensual, material side of life, burning a candle before an image of Venus can be beneficial.

For someone having difficulty with accepting wealth, carrying a tarot card that represents wealth, like the Ten of Pentacles or the Empress, can serve as a point of meditation.

The point here is to track the source of discomfort and move beyond it using magickal means.

Throughout the process of transgressing boundaries, you may also experience guilt. It can be a very difficult emotion to process, and it can be triggered by the smallest things, seemingly out of the blue. Guilt is one of the guardrails that the control society uses to get us to conform to its dictates.

When guilt arises, avoid the tendency to simply give in to it right away. Rather, take the time to investigate the feeling and find its source. Ask yourself if you have really violated some moral precept that matters to you. Oftentimes, you will find you have done nothing wrong in your own judgment, and yet that feeling of guilt is still there. Guilt serves as a reminder of your previous self, before coming out of the closet, before transition, before you chose the path of occult self-empowerment.

In order to sidestep guilt, think of all of the wonderful ways in which you are doing better today than you were when you first embraced your queerness. Record this list of progress in your magickal journal. Examples might include making new friends and acquaintances, being more free to express your fashion choices, feeling more comfortable in your own skin, feeling newfound peace of mind and mental freedom, getting the transition care that you need, etc.

Decorate your list with artwork and poetry. Then, when you are ready, say an affirmation for yourself. It might go something like this: "I set aside my old life with its problems and snares. I awaken to the new life that life has in store for me. I let go of all of the guilt, regret, and shame. My life is becoming new for me. All things are becoming new. All good things come to me today. My path unfolds for me with a steady, smooth direction." When you are done with your affirmation, lightly anoint your magickal record with Florida water or an essential oil.[7] Breathe in the new peace of mind as you let go of the guilt that held you back.

Step 5: Magickal Squares

When you seek to live into your true will, you will face the obstacle of self-defeating, quarreling voices coming from within you, from remnants of past trauma. Some voices will always say, "You are not good enough. Your work is absolute trash. No one will ever accept you." These counter-forces—allegorically encountered as demons, as anti-muses—must be put to rout in order for the magickal work to progress.

William S. Borroughs says that "writing is about making it happen," and this saying can be taken on many levels. On a mundane level, the writer must simply get the fucking work done. This means ignoring all of the naysaying voices, leaping over them, and just getting words on the page. But on another level? We can understand this saying to mean that words have an incantatory or magickal effect.

Brion Gysin, Borroughs's confidant and a visual artist, made works that also functioned as magickal squares or talismans. In this sense, writing (or other creative work) actually brings about changes in the world. Writing makes things happen as reality bends toward the words and the words bend towards reality. Observing the world changes it.

7 Florida water is a light American eau de cologne, with a floral or citrusy scent, used in cleansing and protection rituals.

One way to enter into this sort of work is to make a magickal square (like Gysin), which can function as a sigil. To write a magickal square, simply think of a phrase that encapsulates the work you wish to have happen. This could be something like "finish writing project," "save five hundred dollars," or "get a promotion at work." Then take the phrase and write it in longhand without any spaces or gaps.

Keep writing the phrase until the shape you have created is roughly a square. Then turn the paper 180 degrees and write the same phrase in a perpendicular direction, exactly overlapping what you have just done.

By the time you have finished writing, your magickal square will look like a visually interesting shape that is basically unreadable. Keep it in your magickal journal, on a separate paper, or underneath your pillow until your vision comes true. This will be a very simple way to find success in life and beat some of the mental demons that hold you back from your true will.

Step 6: Asemic and Automatic Writing Experiments

Once you have tried writing magickal squares in words and phrases, you might try asemic writing, which is just using abstract, text-like forms that look aesthetically interesting without conveying determinate meanings. This can be very similar to automatic writing, where you put your mind into autopilot and let go of the need to create a readable text.

Asemic writing can be beautiful, like calligraphy, but it does not create words in a traditional sense.

Try experimenting with nicer pens and paper, like fountain pens and heavy multimedia paper or watercolor paper. In this way, you can create something beautiful that also helps manifest an effective magickal purpose. The purpose you have in mind does not lie in the writing itself but in your intentions.

Asemic writing can free you from the need to express definitive thoughts and help you to progress in an intuitive direction. Try not to overthink this process. Write in free squiggles and word-like shapes without actually creating traditional writing. Arrange the pseudo-language in such a way that it appeals to you as you write on the page. Such a practice is worth many experiments, and it can be a magickal process in its own right.

If asemic writing doesn't work for you, try automatic writing. You might start by doing the chaosphere meditation or the qabalistic cross exercise. Then, take a few minutes to sit calmly with a pen or pencil and close your eyes. Think of a question you would like to have answered. You may feel something beginning to happen, like random scribbles on the page, or you may feel words beginning to form. Try to keep writing until the impulse passes.

Avoid the temptation to control or edit the writing. Just allow the writing to unfold naturally. You may also ask questions as the writing proceeds.

If nothing happens, try coming back to the page again later. Sometimes it can be good to write just before waking or going to sleep, when you are in a more suggestive state of mind. This can be a good way to cut through creative blocks or practice divination.

The most important aspect of automatic writing is to turn off your internal filter, and let yourself go, almost as if you were having an interesting dream. Don't worry about trying to decipher the writing in the moment.

Try coming back to the automatic writing later in much the same way that you would unscramble a puzzle in the morning paper. In time, you may be able to discern different personalities or entities operating in the writing, in a similar way to mediumship.

With automatic writing, you will find that if you relax your hand too much, you will fall into asemic writing that is completely unreadable. But somewhere between a completely relaxed hand and a very tight grip is the right place on the continuum for automatic writing, which can be practiced without the influence of any substances, in ordinary daylight, although proximity to sleep can sometimes be beneficial.

Think of automatic writing as talking to an imaginary friend, a guardian angel, or a kindly spirit that happens to be in the vicinity. Don't worry about writing legibly: just try to get the words onto paper and worry about deciphering later. Your experiments may turn up interesting writing that pertains to what you are doing, whether for a mundane or magickal purpose.

One of my experiments led to the following lines in three short sessions:

1. I am S., the one who wills only your good. Those who read this book will be eloquent and kind. Every person who gets very far in this material will have brushes with occult and . . . experience. You will gather around yourself like minds for the trying and testing of astral ideas. The work does not stop when the book is done. Every person calls to herself laughter for the next generation. You hold to that discursive and and . . . as of plans coming together, plank by plank. But things don't work that way here. We tend to think of everything occurring in the same place and time. We have no waiting until or seeing how things will work out . . .
2. Go up and make a place for yourself. If you can think of calm and peace in your mind, you can also make it real in your life. You have come to this place by many trying and difficult roads. And you do prepare a place for those who come after. Only look after your mind. Take care. Take care. There is only one danger for one who stands apart, who calls great attention. In the recesses and shadows lies the place of power . . . shelter from the storm of life with what may spread powers of time only the powers of your mind that you feel most comfortable with you bring your great contentment.

3. Make many different refinings of . . . so that each and every person who reads these lines will have questions answered. The [raging? nagging?] doubts will fade. It pleases me to make answers plain. It pleases me that [. . .] should be enough. More along for something both or more delightful. Now is the acceptable hour. Now is the time. I am opening the storehouses of wisdom. I am opening the inner sanctum. And there all shall meet and be known.

Most of the illegible text has been removed, and it has been cleaned up a bit. I take it that S. amounts to a familiar spirit who participates in the unfolding of queer magick, as a kind of helper along the way.

In the above lines, we gather important help and advice. It is important for queer mages to keep to inner and outer peace, to try to maintain a stable and supportive world. The original TOPY members kept a room in the house called the nursery, where they would make sigils, and I find this parental feeling apt. If we want our magick to be a support for us, we also have to support our magick, by giving it kind and loving attention.

Or in a romantic relationship, you must talk to your lover, bring them flowers and sweets, and always be on the lookout for their feelings. And so it is with magick. You have to tend your practice, look out for it, and bring gifts to your inner muses. If you "prepare a place" for your magick in your life, it will look out for you in turn.

The second piece of advice that comes out of this automatic writing is that "there is only . . . danger for one who stands apart, who calls great attention." I take this to mean that the practice of magick requires a certain amount of circumspection. It will do no good to try to persuade skeptics, since they likely argue in bad faith and no amount of evidence would convince them anyway. You don't have to take a vow of silence or engage in cloak and dagger theatrics, but it can be better to just keep quiet about the practices you are doing and the results that you have received, at least when it comes to the uninitiated. You definitely want to avoid anyone who would scoff at your spiritual practices or make you feel bad for engaging in occult activity.

Finally, there is a great deal in this automatic writing about spiritual community and handing down the practices to the next generation. Just as there are some people who would be detrimental to your magickal practice, there are others with whom you can and should share your experience, so that you can build yourself some queer magickal community. The inner sanctum is a circle of love and trust that can only be entered by those who share the same goal of advancing along the magickal path together in queer community. With such trusted friends and lovers, you will be able to progress more quickly as you share resources and compare results.

Beyond Control

In this chapter, you learned to fight against the control society that seeks to take away your queerness and uniqueness.

You learned magickal techniques to evoke chaos in your place of work, in order to escape from the confines of drab routines. You also learned a portable method of planetary divination that you can use anytime to get a quick read on a situation. Beyond that, you learned several methods of writing magick, including the making of magickal squares, creating asemic writing, and performing automatic writing.

You also gained some counsel for your magickal practice, learning to be careful about sharing your craft with just anyone. You began thinking about magickal community and the possibility of finding supportive friends and lovers who may be your future partners along the path. You began thinking about the inner sanctum of the Craft, the queer community of those who share this journey with you.

In the days ahead, you will practice the techniques in this chapter many times over, and you will learn to quickly analyze any situation with a planetary reading or just your own intuition. You are to be congratulated on your journey thus far into the chaosphere, and many more adventures await in the pages ahead.

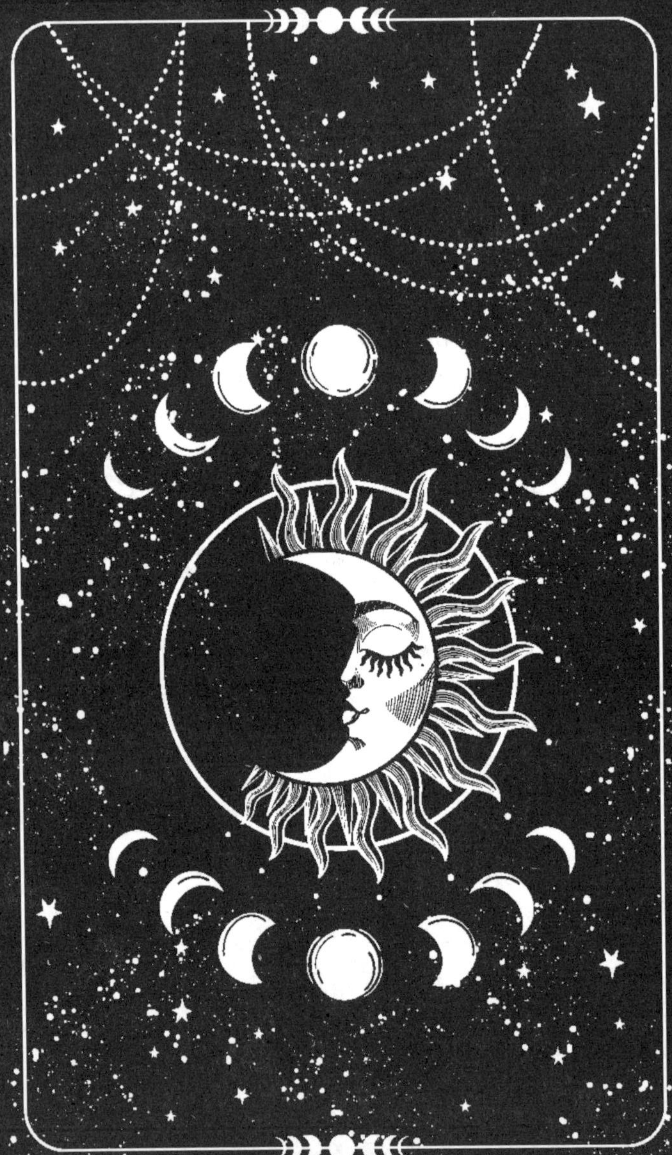

Chapter 6: Inner Vision—Scrying, Visualizing, and Telepathy

What stands between you and your true will? Through the occult tools of scrying, visualization, and telepathy, you can access inner vision and bypass obstacles to the manifestation of your will. When you have finished this chapter, you will have tools at your disposal to work through problems and find solutions to any difficulty.

Chaos magick has a kinship with the universe itself. Almost everything in life changes sooner or later—the job you thought you would have forever, the relationship with the person you thought was your soul mate, the house that you thought would be yours until the end. It's always the end of something. Tragically, comically, or otherwise, all good and bad things come to an end. Our lives are subjected to breakages and ruptures, tragedies and finalities.

But getting comfortable with chaos does not mean shutting off your emotions or trying to avoid getting hurt. At its best, chaos magick should teach us to live deeply and feel every possible emotion on the spectrum. It should allow us our highest highs and lowest lows.

But chaos magick does not mean simply getting comfortable with change or acquiescing to it. Chaos magick should also be about changing the world in conformity with will, taking some of that wild energy of the universe and putting it to work for our own good.

We don't just live in chaos; we also use chaos to secure our own true desires. We are not just flotsam and jetsam in the maelstrom—we are also capable of steering our own way through the storm. No one has absolute freedom, but we can gain a measure of control over fate, destiny, or whatever you want to call it.

That promise of change led you to magick in the first place, and the desire for real change should be the north star of your practice. Every time you open your magickal record, take the time to remember why you were drawn to magick and what you hope to get out of it.

Perhaps you began to practice magick out of a desire for more money or a new career, or maybe you wanted to attract love or sex. Perhaps you were seeking spiritual enlightenment or physical or mental healing.

Always return to that purpose, and remind yourself of it several times a day. It's that inner vision that will guide you through the chaos.

Now we embark on steps that will help you on the journey of connecting to your inner vision.

Step 1: One Month of Intention—A Rededication

Somewhere in your magickal journal, keep for yourself a statement of intention that you can repeat often. You can write your own text or use something like the following:

"I dedicate myself to the wyrding path of change in reliance upon my queer will and my attunement with the chaotic universe. I bind myself, body, mind, and spirit, to fulfilling my aim this day and every day. I will use all magickal and mundane efforts to secure my goal, stopping at nothing until I am well and truly satisfied. I call upon all friendly mortals, gods, and spirits to assist me in my venture. In return, I promise all of my labor to enliven my aim, and I swear my assistance to those who are new to the Craft. I bind to myself all of the fruits of this work, and I pledge myself to be ever alert and active until its completion."

Take the pledge, write it by hand, sign and date it. Read it daily for at least thirty days, and, as you read, hold your purpose firmly in mind. Try repeating the statement when you first rise in the morning, at noon or afternoon, and just before bed.

It becomes especially important to repeat the statement when you are feeling mentally down or weak. If you should feel discouraged or despondent, take a few minutes to yourself and repeat your vow. Purposefully move your emotions to a more positive state. It's important to act "as if" you feel uplifted, encouraged, and strengthened. By acting "as if" you have the desired state, you will come to actually possess it.

By repeating the statement for thirty days, it should be familiar enough to become part of your mental landscape, an enduring testament to the power of your will.

And as you are going through your month, make note in your magickal journal of even the smallest form of assistance that comes to you. For example, if you have been performing work for finding a new job, make note of every resume sent, every phone interview achieved, etc. Make sure to record these as a result of your work. Keep track of all magickal means you have taken as well, such as the use of sigils, visualization, and meditation.

By the end of the month, you should begin to see at least some signs of movement towards your goal. Of course, the bigger the challenge, the more effort will be needed to catalyze the process.

By the end of the month, you will most likely want to keep going with your practice, because it simply feels better internally to be working towards a goal that you find to be personally meaningful.

In the event that your goal has already been completed, start the process again with something a bit more difficult. By way of thanksgiving, you may want to pay your gratitude forward by assisting someone who is new to the Craft, perhaps buying them a new book or some altar candles. If you used any theistic prayers, it is fully appropriate to honor the deities concerned with the appropriate rituals.

Step 2: Scrying with a Pendulum–Thinking, Feeling, and Action

Scrying with a pendulum can be an excellent way to connect with your inner vision.

To begin, draw a triangle inscribed inside of a circle. The three sides of the triangle represent the three faculties of thinking, feeling, and action. Label them.

Make a point at the center of the triangle. The point represents focused desire, the will coming together as one.

For any aim you might wish to achieve, the triangle inscribed inside of a circle represents the forces that you have brought to bear on the situation. Notice that each element must come together perfectly, or the triangle will exceed the bounds of the circle. Just a little bit off in any direction, and the shape will be ruined. This thaumaturgic triangle can be used to diagnose problems with any undertaking, and it can also be used to balance contrary forces and set new projects into motion.

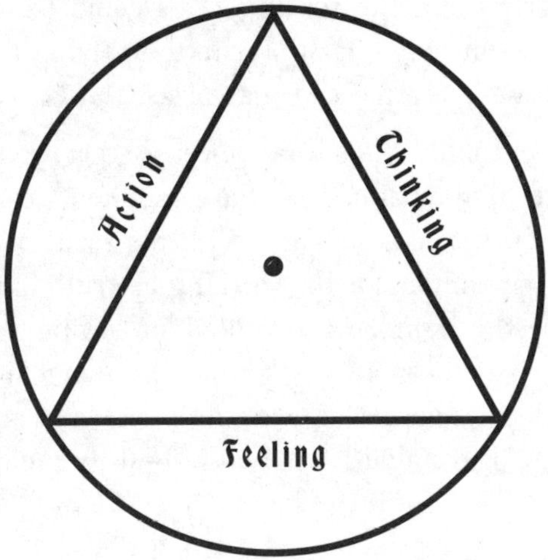

A diagram of a thaumaturgic triangle

Suspend a pendulum above the point in the center of the thaumaturgic triangle. Now you may ask questions pertaining to your aim. An upward pointing triangle has more of a fire orientation, while a downward facing triangle has a water orientation. Use the element most appropriate to your question. You may also choose earth or air by modifying the symbol slightly.[8]

Traditionally, fire governs passion and action, water relates to romance and relationships, air indicates intellect and research, while earth signifies career and finances. By dedicating your divination to the specific element, you make more precise information available.

Begin by holding in mind the aim about which you wish to inquire. See in your mind's eye the undertaking for which you are performing the reading. This could be anything from asking someone out on a date to applying for a new job to creating a new piece of artwork.

Light a candle and some incense that you feel is appropriate to your aim. Pass the pendulum through the smoke of the incense, saying, "With the scent of ____, I purify this pendulum, for the working of truth in my life." Then shine the light on the pendulum, saying, "I invoke the light of truth on this pendulum, so that I may walk with clarity and purpose." Take a drop of water and touch the triangle diagram with it, saying, "I purify the threefold inner vision."

---

8 The alchemical symbol for air is an equilateral triangle with a horizontal bar through it. Earth is an inverted equilateral triangle with a line through it. These symbols can be easily found online.

Now you are in a position to enter into a dialogue with the pendulum. In general, if the pendulum moves towards the top of the diagram, this can be equated with yes. If the pendulum moves towards the bottom of the diagram, this can be equated with no. A clockwise direction of travel indicates things, people, and resources being drawn into your life, while a counterclockwise direction of travel indicates things, people, and resources leaving your life. If the pendulum stays near the center, this indicates a calm, clear situation without a lot of dynamism. If the pendulum is moving around all over the place, you have a very dynamic situation with a lot of change and a lot of players.

Take into account the three areas of thinking, feeling, and acting. You might ask the pendulum, "What is my greatest area of strength for this undertaking?" If the pendulum goes toward action, the reading is telling you that you are a very proactive person, that you have not been afraid to take charge of the situation, and that your initiative works in your favor. If it goes toward feeling, the pendulum is telling you that you have been very empathetic in this situation, that you have a lot of emotional maturity and insight. If it goes towards thinking, the pendulum is telling you that you have spent a lot of time analyzing the situation from all angles, that you have a good understanding of the dynamics at work.

In terms of the weaknesses of the three areas, if you are deficient in action, your plans will not come together no matter how well-considered they are. Weakness in action can only be remedied by taking a chance on a situation, even if the circumstances are not perfect. If you are deficient in feeling, you may accomplish your aim at the cost of important relationships in your life. The pendulum may be telling you to exercise care with the emotions of the people close to you. If you are deficient in thinking, the pendulum is telling you that you have not spent the proper amount of time in planning for your use of resources. You may need to spend more time just writing down the steps of your plan or estimating your budget.

You can enter into dialogue with the pendulum for as long as you like. By asking yes-or-no questions, or thinking-feeling-acting questions, you can get a pretty comprehensive picture of the situation.

You can even use the pendulum to do custom readings for questions like, "Who is my biggest supporter at work?" or "What day of this week will be the best for making sigils?" In the case of custom questions, you can just write on a piece of paper the available choices and allow the pendulum to guide you to the appropriate answer.

As you work with the pendulum, you may sometimes wonder if you are being guided by the pendulum or if you are guiding it to say what you already wanted it to say. Approach the scrying with an inner intensity, in a spirit of simply wanting to get down to the truth of the matter. If you approach the pendulum with sincerity and faith, you will feel a kind of guiding force pushing back against your desires. In other words, it will feel like someone else is there with you, guiding you into receiving the knowledge that you desire.

When it comes time to close your session, say a few words in closing, like, "I give thanks to the spirit of this time and place, for the guidance and direction received here today. I promise to follow through on all of the insights gained here, and I promise to share the light that I have seen."

Keep your pendulum in a safe place, preferably in your altar area or around crystals where it can receive positive vibrations. The pendulum can be charged in much the same way as a crystal, by placing it in sunlight or moonlight.

Step 3: Finding Your Inner Oasis

Sometimes you may be in need of rest or advice on your journey with inner vision and queer chaos magick. As you face a queerphobic world, you might need a place to get away from it all and in touch with your intuition. This exercise, really a guided visualization, can provide you with a home away from home, a sanctuary within your own mind that you can visit whenever you like. I made this inner oasis a farmhouse, because I like to return to my maternal grandparents' house in my mind's eye. You can feel free to alter the experience however you like.

Get as comfortable as you can, preferably lying down on your bed or on a yoga mat. Begin by visualizing the color red. Make the color red as intense as you can imagine. If you have trouble with this, imagine a red tomato, a red fire engine, a red dress. Hold the color red in your mind's eye.

And then shift to the color orange, a vibrant, brilliant orange. Make the orange as bright as you can, and allow it to fill your visual field. With each color, you are moving deeper into your own subconscious mind.

And next, visualize the color yellow, a bright yellow, like a lemon. And allow the yellow to grow more intense and fill your interior landscape. The color yellow is taking you deeper into your subconscious mind. You feel incredibly calm and relaxed.

Next the color yellow begins to morph into green, first a light spring green and then a deeper Kelly green. The intense green color fills your field of vision, so that you can only see green, all around. The color green is taking you deeper into your subconscious mind.

And next comes the color blue. Visualize the color blue. The color blue deepens and intensifies. The color blue takes you deeper into your subconscious mind.

And blue gives way to indigo, a deeper, more intense shade.

Finally, indigo gives way to violet. You are surrounded by a violet light, around you and through you. You can see yourself in your mind's eye, surrounded by a cloud of violet light.

Violet gives way to a brilliant white light. You see yourself standing in a white hallway. The walls are white, the floor is white, and the ceiling is white. You take a few steps down this white hallway. And you see yourself reaching a stairwell leading down. You know that the stairwell has ten steps.

As you go down each step, you move further into your subconscious mind. You are deeply in touch with your inner spirit, with your inner intuition, with the deepest part of who you are. And very slowly, you begin by stepping down to the tenth step.

Very gently and intentionally you step down to the ninth step. Moving deeper and deeper into your subconscious mind.

And stepping down to the eighth step. Deeper still into your own heart, your own spirit.

Stepping down to the seventh step. And you are twice as deep as you were before.

And on to the sixth step, getting calmer and more relaxed.

Now, you step down to the fifth step. And now, you are moving deeper and deeper into your subconscious mind.

You step down to the fourth step. You are deep into a dream-like state, a trance state of mind.

And you step down to the third step. You are feeling so comfortably relaxed. You are not sure if you have ever felt this relaxed before.

And down to the second step. Finally down to the first step. And you are at the bottom of the stairs.

You take a few steps forward, and in front of you, you see a doorway. You can make the doorway any style or material that you like. Feel free to make it your own, make it unique. You reach out and grab the door knob, and it turns. You find yourself stepping outside.

The doorway opens onto the countryside. The wind is blowing in the trees, there are green fields all around. You can hear a stream somewhere nearby. Birds are singing in the trees. You walk forward over a little hill, and just there over the hill, you find a dirt or gravel pathway. Following the pathway, you see that it leads past some fields where crops are growing, perhaps some herbs or vegetables.

Finally, you come to a gate with a latch. You open the latch and go inside, down a small footpath with stepping stones. And the stepping stones lead to a porch surrounding a farmhouse. You see on the broad porch a place with a bench where you can take off your shoes, and there is a table here as well. You take off your shoes and sit at the table.

There is someone sitting here at the table with you, one of the people who lives in the farmhouse. Here you will pause for your first conversation. Introduce yourself to this person, and find out their name as well. They may give you a job to do, like shelling peas or folding clothes, and the two of you will have a little chat. Imagine that you are talking with someone who is very practical but also wise. Now is the chance to ask any questions that you might have and to begin a relationship with a familiar spirit. Every time you come back here, this person will be here, on the porch, always ready for a chat.

And when you are ready, you can knock on the door to the farmhouse proper. A second person, a second spirit will answer the door. Again, you are meeting someone incredibly wise who cares about you and any problems or questions that you might have. This person will be your host throughout the rest of the session. Make sure to introduce yourself and get their name as well. Remember it for the next time that you return.

Your host greets you and ushers you into a large living room. You sit on a cushion on the floor, and your host brings you something to drink. You are now prepared to ask a question, any possible question that you can imagine. There is nothing too simple or too difficult for this place. Anything you might want to know is within bounds.

Your host has you think of an object to represent your question. For example, a question about your finances might be represented by a checkbook or a debit card. A question about work might be represented by your name tag. A spiritual question could be represented by a mala or a medallion of some kind. You will think of this object and place it in a tray that the host provides. It may transform as it goes into the tray. For example, it may turn to brass or become more ornamental.Your host asks you to call witnesses to answer your question. These witnesses may be living or dead or even mythological. You can call your grandmother, Socrates, or the Buddha. This is a completely private conversation for your benefit alone. This conversation is for you and your clearness of mind. You call your witnesses, and they enter the room and sit in a circle.

You pass your ceremonial object around the room, so that it becomes a talking stick. Each person in the room will have an opportunity to answer your question. The session ends when everyone has had a chance to speak.

After everyone has spoken, make sure to thank each of your witnesses for attending the session, as well as your hosts at the farmhouse. When you are finished, you may walk back outside and reverse the steps that you took to get here. Or you may simply open your eyes and return to everyday life.

Note that this procedure can be used for many different purposes. You can ask for life advice about any problems that might be bothering you. You can ask for ritual advice about how to make your sigils and spells more effective. You can even ask bigger questions, like how to bring about world peace or how to find enlightenment.

The answers that you receive will be unique to you as an individual and personalized to your exact life situation at the time of the reading. Just be sure to do this practice regularly. Think about it like you are forming a relationship with your familiar spirits. They will worry about you when they do not see you, and they are always happy to hear your voice. Treat these relationships with a degree of responsibility, like you would do with people in the regular world. The more you nurture these relationships, the more they will support you.

Over time, you will begin to explore the world of the farmhouse in greater detail. You may use other rooms of the house for different purposes. Maybe you actually conduct rituals inside one of the rooms of the farmhouse. You may discover other structures, like the potting shed or other outbuildings, which have their own purposes. The world of the farmhouse will become more detailed and complex with time, and you will meet many other spirits who help to tend the place and keep it habitable. As long as you are kind and respectful in your dealings, you will continue to gain many insights through this meditative space.

Step 4: Dream Telepathy

As a queer person and a chaos magician, you may often find yourself at odds with mainstream society. You have a personal and artistic vision that you long to express in the world. You are not content with simply surviving or getting by. You have definite goals you would like to achieve in life.

Maybe you would like to be able to earn a living with writing or artwork. Maybe you would like to be able to move in with your partner or buy a home. Maybe you would like to pursue an activism project or start a nonprofit.

The good news? You can use your magickal pathway to catalyze the life of your dreams, especially in times where you may be feeling stuck or blocked in some way.

Some of the most interesting things happen in the borderline between wakefulness and sleep, or during the times when we are actually asleep and dreaming. We can make use of our dream times and actually use sleep to cast spells that will lead to our greater peace of mind and well-being.

As Mitch Horowitz, historian of alternative spirituality, explains in *The Miracle Club: How Thoughts Become Reality,* we can begin by creating a scene in our minds that implies the fulfillment of some deeply held goal. If you are seeking employment, for example, you might imagine yourself receiving a handshake upon being offered the job. Or you might imagine getting that first paycheck in the mail. It is important to build into this mental scene as much emotional connection as possible. Feel the happiness and satisfaction that goes along with this scene while you visualize it.

As you lay down to sleep at night, put away your phone and any other distractions. Lay down and close your eyes. Then, play your scene of success over and over again in your mind's eye. See yourself getting the job, closing on a house, or starting your nonprofit—whatever your success story may be. Picture the success as already accomplished, as though you have already received the thing you want. Drift off to sleep while you are having this vision of accomplishment.

When you wake the next morning, try to remember any dreams you had. Write down an account of your dreams using as much detail as possible. Then take the resulting description and make a sigil using the cut-up method. Your subconscious mind will be put to work fulfilling your aim, and the resulting sigil will become a concretization of your desire.

When you have tried this by yourself, try working with a partner, someone you know and trust. Share with your partner the reason why you want to do the undertaking, and your partner will share with you as well. Agree on a night to do the practice. Ideally, it should be a time when you know you will be able to get plenty of rest, and the following day is not too stressful. If you like, you can take into account the phases of the moon, using a waxing to full moon for constructive work and a waning to new moon for cleansing, banishing work. Check in with your partner just before bed. Agree that you will try to remember your dreams and share them with each other the next day.

On the following morning, both you and your partner will write down your dreams and share the transcripts. This can be an interesting exercise in its own right; you may see a tendency of the dreams to converge with one another. Then, you will have two texts—one of your dream and one of your partner's. These two texts can be cut-up and reassembled into one magickal sigil to accomplish your aims. The two of you will become co-conspirators in the work. The magickal working can become the basis for other forms of partnership as you offer each other material assistance in reaching the life of your dreams.

It takes a good deal of vulnerability to be able to open yourself to working magickally with someone. This kind of openness goes against the grain of our culture, where, as Westerners, we often think we have to go it alone and do everything by ourselves.

Opening our minds and hearts to others acknowledges our dependence on factors greater than ourselves, our reliance upon the higher mind of nature, the greater expansiveness of all of our work. This greater mind influences all that we do, and through it, we have connection to one another, even when we are not communicating in words. Dream telepathy works through this invisible medium, and this higher mind also enables the Craft of magick to function. Without the higher mind of nature, we would all be essentially stuck in our separate worlds, unable to connect with any reality beyond ourselves.

Step 5: Tarot of Endings and Death

When you did the dream telepathy exercise, you committed yourself to a vision of something you deeply want. You made a sigil to express your desire to have some sort of transformation take place in your life. At this point, you are willing to do anything to have your vision become a reality. Now, you will take a look at the flipside of your vision, in terms of some of the habits of mind that may be holding you back from getting what you want. In other words, there are things in your life that need to be gone and done in order for your desire to become a reality.To complete this exercise, draw a tarot trump that has to do with endings and conclusions. I am thinking specifically of Death, the Tower, Judgment, and the World. Take a look at these four cards and see if one of them speaks to you on a deeper level. Spend some time just meditating on the image and seeing what it says to you. Light a candle so that it illuminates the card you have chosen, and keep gazing upon it until you know it by heart.

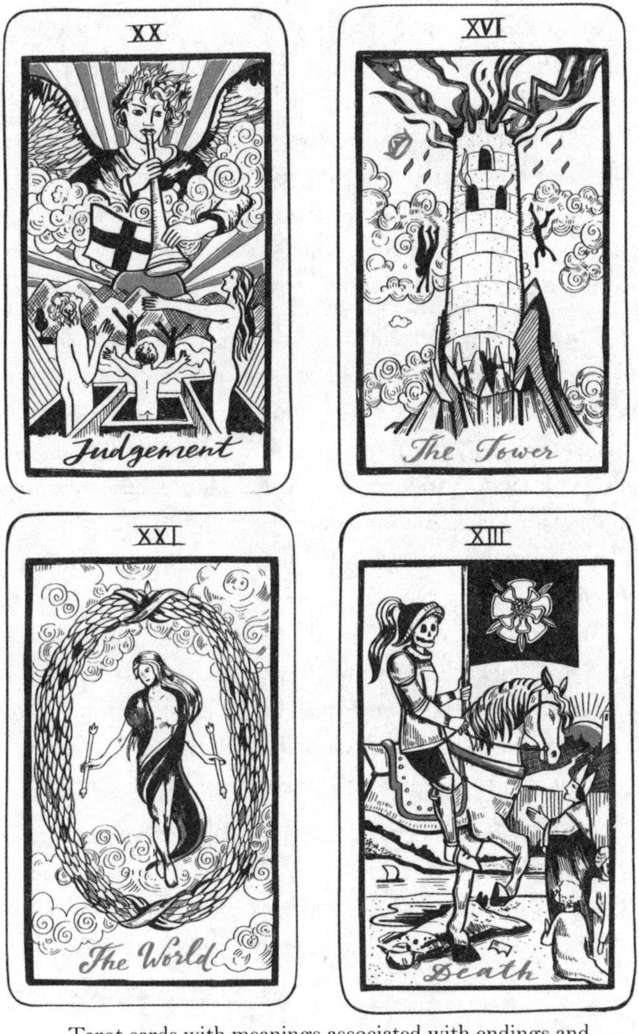

Tarot cards with meanings associated with endings and conclusions: Death, the Tower, Judgment, and the World.

When you have internalized the card thoroughly, take a scrap piece of paper and begin writing down the things that hold you back from getting what you want. Begin with habits of the mind. Perhaps you have a habit of self-doubt that causes you to feel unworthy. Maybe you experienced some hardship in your early life that makes you feel like you are not as valuable as other people. Maybe you tend to self-sabotage by not working up to your full potential. Maybe you have some internalized transphobia or homophobia that makes you feel inferior to those around you. Write down a candid description of your particular obstacle.

Now move to relationships you know have some sort of problematic aspect. There may be someone in your life who subjects you to subtle or not-so-subtle put-downs, who makes you feel bad about yourself. There may be someone at work who undermines you, like a micromanaging supervisor or someone who takes credit for your work. There may be relationships with service providers, like physicians or therapists, that don't seem to be functioning the way they should. Take the time to describe exactly the way that the relationship does not serve you. Right now, you need not devote any time to solutions—limit yourself to describing the aspects of the relationship that are not helping you to reach your goals.

Finally, consider the material reality of your life and the ways that it does not serve you. Perhaps your physical space is so small you don't have room to undertake your artwork. Maybe you don't have the startup funds you need to begin your new venture. Maybe you lack the time necessary to make your project a reality. Spend a few minutes describing, in detail, all of the limiting factors holding you back.

Now, you should have down on paper a description of all of the bad habits, the broken relationships, and the meager circumstances that hold you back from living the life of your dreams. While holding a vision of your chosen tarot card in your mind, burn your piece of writing in an unconsecrated fire. Watch the flames devour all of the factors that hold you back in life. While the fire is burning, will yourself be done with all of these limiting beliefs, relationships, and circumstances.

You may feel the need to let out a sigh or a groan as you do this, as you are well and truly letting go of what has held you back for so long. Truly believe in your mind and heart that you are making a change that will make a tremendous difference for you going forward.

As optional steps, you might consider tying a piece of black string around one wrist as a way to remind yourself of the real commitment that you have made to change. Keep wearing the thread until it falls off your wrist as a reminder of the changes that you will see coming into your life.

Another thing you might do as a reminder is to keep returning to the tarot card you selected. Every time you gaze upon the card, you symbolically rekindle the cleansing fire that takes away the negative forces from your life.

As another action step, you might make your own version of the card that you selected. You might try collage, painting, or drawing. Artwork is a great way to internalize the meaning of the card and make it personal to yourself.

A Refuge and Strength

In this chapter, you rededicated yourself to fulfilling your true will and set down on paper your commitment to living the life of your dreams. You learned to use a pendulum to ask questions about thinking, feeling, and action, finding insight into your areas of weakness and strength. You learned to use the farmhouse exercise to find answers to the pressing questions that you have about your life's journey. You used dream telepathy to create a magickal spell to fulfill your heart's desire, and you used the tarot to clear away obstacles blocking your path.

You have just learned many skills for your life journey to peace and empowerment. The exercises in this chapter improve with age; they are to be repeated many times over, so that you mature in your understanding of your path. With time, you will grow more firm in your commitment to the life that you want, and you will better be able to set boundaries and say no to what does not serve you.

As this book draws to a close, we will look closer at chaos as a personified force. We will learn how to draw closer to chaos and enter into a relationship with it. We will further dispel any fear about the uncertainty that the future holds, and we will learn to use chaos as a factor in our favor as we move deeper into the chaosphere.

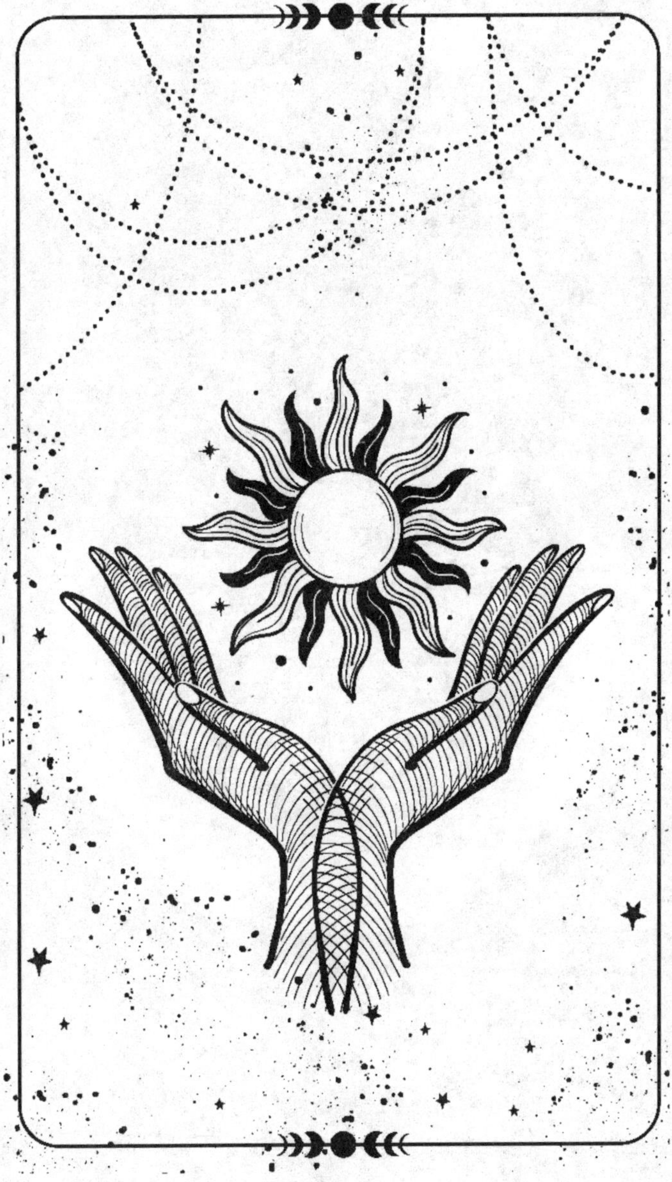

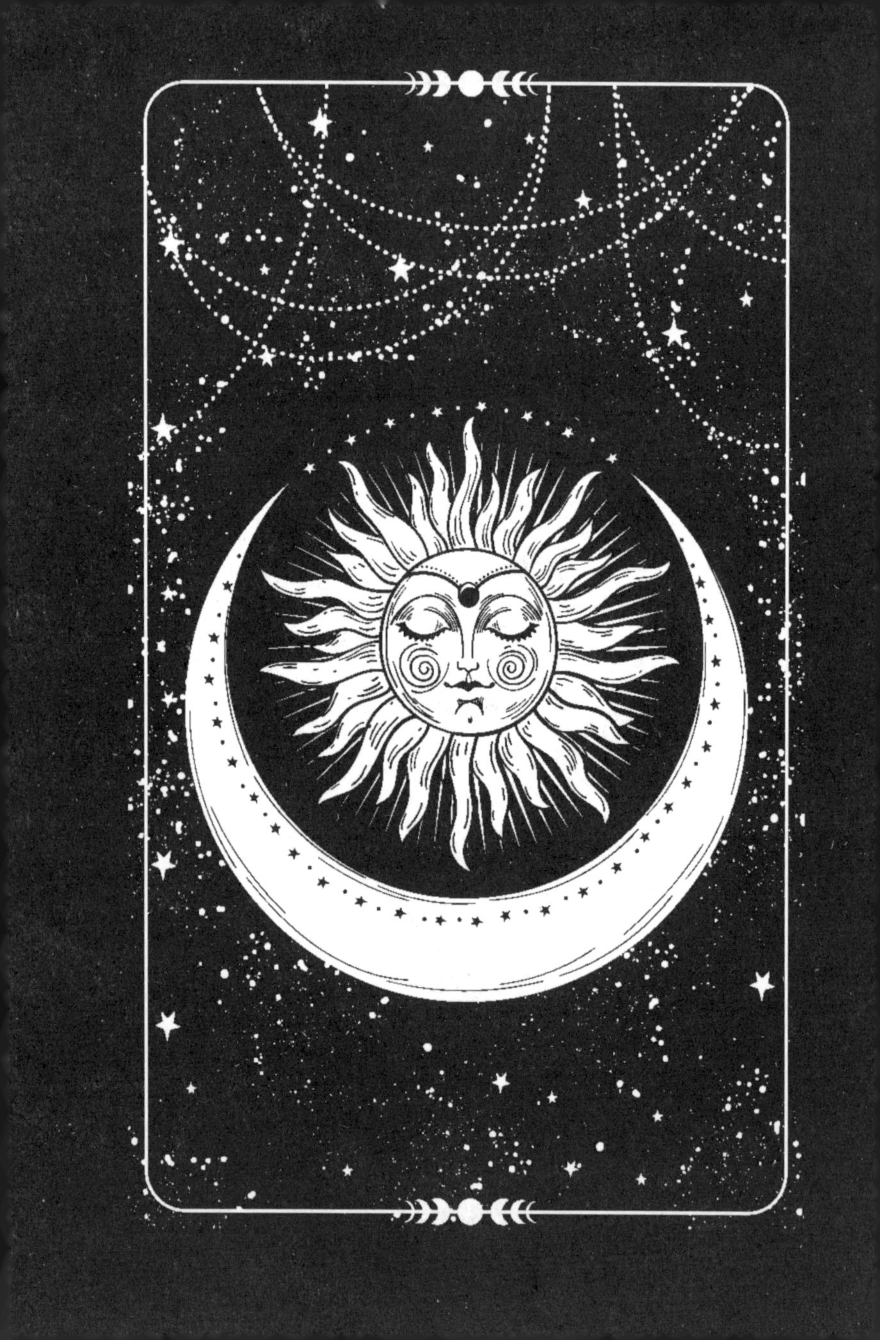

Chapter 7: Invoking Chaos

Chaos need not be avoided or controlled: it can be actively invoked to bring the power of change into your life. The invocation of chaos brings raw, transformative energy as you chant its names and stare into its broken mirror.

Invoking chaos need not be difficult or distressing, as the step-by-step instructions in this chapter will make you able to perform the ritual with minimal materials. And thus, chaos as a change agent will enter your life to undo tired assumptions and bring fresh new realities into being.

By the end of this chapter, you will know how to invoke chaos, how to conduct broken mirror scrying, and how to bring spontaneity into your life.

No matter how much positive thinking you do or how many mantras you say, life is still hard. You have to contend not only with the laws of physics but also with the economic and political realities of our times.

It can be difficult living as a queer magician in the world today, in times that do not feel very friendly to LGBTQIA+ people. So often legislators seek to erase our very existence through bans on gender-affirming care, bans on LGBTQIA+ books in schools, bans on trans athletes, and other bans on vital aspects of our community. And then there are the everyday difficulties of paying rent, buying groceries, and paying the bills.

When it feels like everything is going wrong, like the world is falling apart around you, it can be hard to muster the energy to work on spells or practice divination. It can be hard to muster the positive frame of mind which says yes, change is possible. Fortunately, in chaos we have a mode of magick that is multifaceted, that is not limited to only one practice or set of practices. We can stack the deck of fate by going into chaos directly and becoming one with it. As we enter into chaos, we enter into the heart of the universe itself, and that becomes a powerful source of refuge in turbulent times.

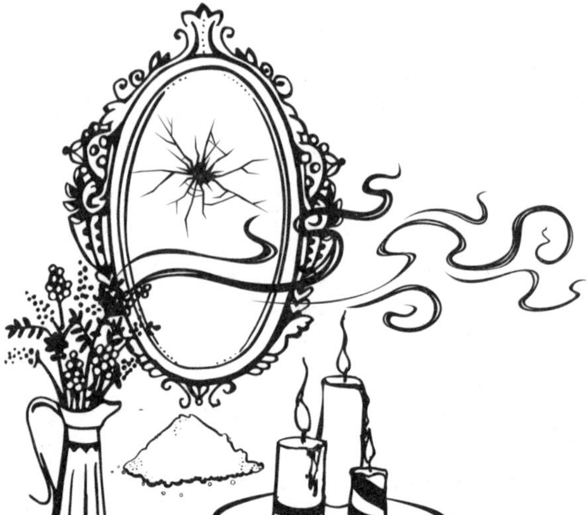

Invoking chaos with a black candle, a broken mirror, a flower, salt, and incense

Chaos is a tendency of magick, a tendency of the world itself, and also one of the oldest divinities in the western world. Hesiod's *Theogony*, composed perhaps in 730 to 700 BCE, has the poet inspired directly by the muses, and naming chaos as the first deity, coming just before the earth, night and day, and the other immortals.

In what follows, you will become more familiar with the names of chaos, as inspired by Greek mythology, with a bit of influence from the *Tao Te Ching* and modern chaos magick. By drawing near to chaos through mystical chanting, you take shelter from this powerful force and make it easier to dwell in our turbulent world.

Step 1: Invocation of Chaos

This slightly longer invocation of chaos can be used as a preliminary to any ritual work. It should be used whenever you need a strong connection to the primal forces of magick. The recitations in this invocation are a way of occupying the mind so that it does not stray, and the ritual elements also help to control the senses. The whole body ultimately becomes absorbed in the ritual action.

The invocation can be performed while seated or standing, but a small table will be necessary for placing the required items. It is also possible to only recite the invocation without the ritual implements. Substitutions may also be made if you lack any of the requisite items.

Begin with the chaosphere meditation discussed in chapter 2. Take your time in visualizing the chaosphere—the cube inscribed inside of a sphere with eight rays going outward toward the corners of the cube. You may also picture a crossroads going in the four cardinal directions. See the sphere, the cube, the rays, and the four roads glowing in a blue-white light.

Then repeat the reflection, as usual: *I dissolve my thoughts into the blue-white light of chaos. I release my thoughts into the All. I dissolve my feelings into the blue-white light of chaos. I release my feelings into the All. I dissolve my actions into the blue-white light of chaos. I release my actions into the All. I have become indifferent to gain and loss. I have become indifferent to pain and pleasure. All roads converge for me in the All. My dream is my destiny and mine alone. I have become chaos, progenitor and destroyer of worlds.*

This time, instead of drawing the chaosphere down the axis of the body, allow it to expand until it is as large as the room you are in. The idea is that the magickal shape maps onto the physical space itself. Endeavor to see the chaosphere in your mind's eye, consecrating the space where you are conducting the ritual work.

Then, proceed as follows, reciting while placing the ritual objects (incense, salt, candle, broken mirror):

I enter into this darkened space consecrated unto you, mother chaos, the most ancient one and first among the gods of old. I come before you as your acolyte to honor you and seek your presence. I put aside all extraneous thoughts and vow to concentrate my mind upon you alone, so that I might seek your company and counsel. I come to you without knowledge of the proper way to receive you. I ask that you overlook the faults in the performance of this ritual and enter into this place today. Make yourself known to me so that I may serve as your vessel.

I burn this smoky incense to remind me of your murky darkness before the foundation of the world. I smell the sweetness of these fragrant resins, which reminds me of your inward and secret presence in all things. (Waft the incense in the four cardinal directions as well as above and below. Place the incense on the altar table.)

I place this salt to remind me of your primeval waters and the churning action of your great power. I taste this salt to remind me of the sweat of my brow, by which you accomplish your great work in the world. (Place the salt on the altar table and taste a small amount of it.)

I light this black candle to remind me of your luminous darkness, the inner wyrding light by which we see the magickal world. I purify myself and this space by means of light. (Shine the light on your own face and on the room and anyone in it.)

I place this broken mirror to remind me that all things reflect your beauty and that you dwell in the fractured places of the world. I see myself in this broken mirror, and my many faces look back at me. (Gaze into the broken mirror, and allow anyone else in the room to do so.)

Now, recite the 108 names of chaos, as follows below. (Optional: Small stones, shells, or other bits of ephemera may be placed with each name.)

1. *Hail chaos, destroyer of worlds.*
2. *Hail chaos, mother of worlds.*
3. *Hail chaos, who is the maelstrom.*
4. *Hail chaos, darkness within darkness.*
5. *Hail chaos, mother of the muses.*
6. *Hail chaos, first of the primordial ones.*
7. *Hail chaos, who surrounds the Earth.*
8. *Hail chaos, mother of heaven.*
9. *Hail chaos, mother of night and day.*
10. *Hail chaos, who is fate and destiny.*
11. *Hail chaos, who protects birds of the air.*
12. *Hail chaos, who is robed with the night.*
13. *Hail chaos, daughter of time.*
14. *Hail chaos, daughter of necessity.*
15. *Hail chaos, the inscrutable one.*
16. *Hail chaos, comfort to the destitute.*
17. *Hail chaos, scourge of the mighty.*
18. *Hail chaos, out of which gods arose.*
19. *Hail chaos, origin of humans and spirits.*
20. *Hail chaos, progenitor of darkness and night.*
21. *Hail chaos, who is the abyss.*
22. *Hail chaos, who is infinite complexity.*
23. *Hail chaos, who cannot be contained.*
24. *Hail chaos, who is nothingness.*
25. *Hail chaos, who is all of existence.*

26. *Hail chaos, who brings panic.*
27. *Hail chaos, who makes things new.*
28. *Hail chaos, source of reality.*
29. *Hail chaos, the formless void.*
30. *Hail chaos, the end of the ages.*
31. *Hail chaos, the beginning of all things.*
32. *Hail chaos, first of the gods.*
33. *Hail chaos, the primordial mud.*
34. *Hail chaos, origin of life.*
35. *Hail chaos, who overthrows all.*
36. *Hail chaos, who is the crossroads.*
37. *Hail chaos, who is entropy.*
38. *Hail chaos, darkness on the face of the waters.*
39. *Hail chaos, who is older than God.*
40. *Hail chaos, who is the All.*
41. *Hail chaos, who contains all.*
42. *Hail chaos, who cannot be known.*
43. *Hail chaos, who is rot and decay.*
44. *Hail chaos, who brings new life.*
45. *Hail chaos, the fabric of the cosmos.*
46. *Hail chaos, who is queer.*
47. *Hail chaos, who devours gods.*
48. *Hail chaos, source of all magick.*
49. *Hail chaos, who is possibility.*
50. *Hail chaos, who is infinitely small.*
51. *Hail chaos, end of all things.*
52. *Hail chaos, container of all.*
53. *Hail chaos, garment of destiny.*

54. Hail chaos, seer of all.

55. Hail chaos, who dwells in the whirlwind.

56. Hail chaos, breaker of chains.

57. Hail chaos, who is at play.

58. Hail chaos, who is ever active.

59. Hail chaos, who remains at rest.

60. Hail chaos, who is nowhere.

61. Hail chaos, who is everywhere.

62. Hail chaos, who was struck by the thunderbolt.

63. Hail chaos, the shapeless one.

64. Hail chaos, origin of earth.

65. Hail chaos, who generates the underworld.

66. Hail chaos, order in disorder.

67. Hail chaos, mother of weirdness.

68. Hail chaos, ceaseless repetition.

69. Hail chaos, absolutely unique.

70. Hail chaos, pattern within the pattern.

71. Hail chaos, who cannot be described.

72. Hail chaos, the smallest of the small.

73. Hail chaos, the immeasurably great.

74. Hail chaos, into whom all things return.

75. Hail chaos, neverending change.

76. Hail chaos, who remains the same.

77. Hail chaos, the nameless one.

78. Hail chaos, who breaks bonds asunder.

79. Hail chaos, who swings the pendulum.

80. Hail chaos, refuge of many.

81. Hail chaos, giver of second sight.

82. *Hail chaos, the eye of the storm.*
83. *Hail chaos, who is unstable.*
84. *Hail chaos, who is reality itself.*
85. *Hail chaos, the most ancient one.*
86. *Hail chaos, the most dependable.*
87. *Hail chaos, the secret of secrets.*
88. *Hail chaos, who cannot be controlled.*
89. *Hail chaos, who brings change.*
90. *Hail chaos, who brings fulfillment.*
91. *Hail chaos, who strengthens the mind.*
92. *Hail chaos, most severe.*
93. *Hail chaos, of infinite mercy.*
94. *Hail chaos, who crushes expectations.*
95. *Hail chaos, who is raven black.*
96. *Hail chaos, who is smoke and ash.*
97. *Hail chaos, the thunderous waters.*
98. *Hail chaos, who lives in all.*
99. *Hail chaos, who is the heartbeat.*
100. *Hail chaos, who is the breath.*
101. *Hail chaos, who is the end.*
102. *Hail chaos, who is close at hand.*
103. *Hail chaos, who remains unknown.*
104. *Hail chaos, the music of the void.*
105. *Hail chaos, who creates variety.*
106. *Hail chaos, the luminous darkness.*
107. *Hail chaos, the mist of forgetting.*
108. *Hail chaos, who is unknowing.*

By means of this rite, I purify this place and my own mind and heart. I invoke the power of chaos into this world for the operation of my will. (Silently state your request here.) *I pledge my effort and will to accomplish the purpose that I have set for myself today. May all of my thoughts bear fruit. May all of my feelings find expression. May all of my actions yield their intended results. I bind myself to the path of chaos today. I see in all things the unfolding of a hidden pattern, by which dark purposes unfold. I will see no obstacle that does not hold an unseen advantage. I bind myself to the accomplishing of my will, no matter what occurs.*

Chaos, dark yawning abyss,

from whom came the worlds and all the gods,

Take me to yourself today.

Hide my words, my will, and my works in your embrace.

May I see by the dark light that you shine on my path.

At this point, gaze once more into the broken mirror. Then, put it away or cover it with a cloth.

Wave your hand through the incense smoke, drawing it toward yourself and over your head, and then extinguish the censer.

Taste the salt once more and then put it away.

Wave your hand over the light and then extinguish it.

If more than one person is participating, everyone should be given an opportunity to gaze in the mirror, taste the salt, wave hands through the smoke, etc.

If at all possible, try not to rush away from the performance of the ritual. Take a few minutes to absorb the atmosphere created by the work. Take note of any insights that come your way and record them in your magickal record.

Step 2: The Power of Possibility

Aligning yourself with chaos—the wild, queer energy at the heart of the universe—means that you are also affirming certain truths about yourself and your own life. The world ceaselessly changes, and with it, your own life and even your own identity.

You may have been weighed down in the past with a feeling of drudgery, like the daily grind would simply devour you whole. You may have had a feeling of almost unbearable tedium, together with a sense of exhaustion at the world's inexorable march towards destruction.

The word *chaos* can be scary, because it implies entropy and disorder, and indeed, the world does exhibit signs of disorder and a great deal of dysfunction as well. But chaos magick is ultimately hopeful, because it suggests that anything you don't like can be changed.

When you invoked chaos in the previous exercise, you gazed into a broken mirror. The broken mirror, of course, symbolizes bad luck. But by intentionally breaking the mirror and gazing into it, you take hold of bad luck and turn it around. You affirm that what seems negative on the outside actually holds transformative potential. The chaos that breaks things and destroys them also recreates and renews. The river that floods the fields is the same river that waters the crops. What tears asunder also makes anew. This rending, scouring action can feel harsh sometimes, as when a job or a relationship ends unexpectedly. But this same chaotic force also brings the potential for positive change.

The mirror also symbolizes narcissism, an over-concentration on outward appearances and an attachment to the ego nature. By breaking the mirror and gazing into it, you affirm that there is not just one solitary self who rules over your life like a despot. Rather, you have many selves, many narratives competing for control.

Some of those selves are shadow selves. Sometimes you hide aspects of yourself, because you fear rejection of that facet of your personality. Maybe you like to compose music, but you fear that no one will like your songs. Or you may suppress your sense of humor, because it feels like it doesn't fit in your professional life. By gazing into the broken mirror, you affirm all of those faces gazing back at you. All of the aspects of your personality are your real self. They all deserve time in the light of day.

The broken mirror also represents all of the relationships in your life. These relationships manifest in fractal patterns of complexity. You may be attracted to women or men or nonbinary people or all of the above. You may have a strong sex drive or be asexual, demisexual, or aromantic. You may have a relatively simple romantic history, or you may have a huge backstory of past liaisons. Some of the relationships in your past may leave only fond memories behind, while others may hold histories of trauma and abuse.

Your mirror work expresses the complexity in your past history, as well as in your gender identity and sexual expression. By gazing into the mirror, you affirm that yes, all those aspects of yourself are there, and yes, they are all real.

The mirror is not just about the past. You also take time during the invocation to speak your requests into the void. But you speak them aloud with the real conviction that your wants and desires matter.

By speaking your requests or by building them into a sigil, you actually broadcast them into the universe. And the universe actually hears what you say in your ritual work. A tiny thought may not seem like it has much power, but it is like the beating of a butterfly's wing that gives rise to the tornado. A small, local change can have a large, nonlinear effect in any complex system. As you conduct the ritual, you reprogram your subconscious mind to believe in the real potential for positive change. And that belief in the power of change actually creates it.

As you work your rituals, the change inherent in the universe will begin to work in your favor. You will begin to see little glimmers of hope. Your friends and colleagues will become more helpful as you seek to fulfill your aims. You will receive little forms of material support—a check will arrive in the mail, a side gig will appear. You will also notice inward changes as you work with the practices in this book; your old despondency will give way to a brighter outlook. Your cynicism will at least occasionally give way to a newfound interest in people and the world. You will begin to see possibility when things seemed hopeless before.

Sometimes you find magick when you have the greatest need of it, when your back is against a wall. Think about the circumstances that led you to magick in the first place. You most likely felt some sort of lack in your life, some desire for more of something—more love, more money, more power, etc.

And chaos magick is not here to tell you that you are wrong to want what you want, because magick is about life. And life is about the desire for more. Life continuously seeks to exceed its old boundaries, like the sapling growing up toward the light or the snake shedding its skin.

So do not be ashamed of wanting what you want, and speak your desires. Speaking them aloud, if only to yourself, is the first step to getting what you want.

Step 3: Fulfilling the Promise

Magick should be about making your life bigger, bolder, and better than ever before. It should be about transformation of your latent potential, helping you to metamorphosize into the person you were meant to become. And it should be results-oriented.

If you do not see progress along the path, magick is just an entertaining diversion. To that end, magick should help you develop for yourself a clear picture of who you are and who you want to become. You have already developed this picture to a large degree. You already know that you are a queer person who practices chaos magick. You probably know a great many other things about yourself as well. Some of the exercises in this book have helped you to clarify your past, present, and future selves.

Now it is time to do some more visioning in concrete terms about your life and your hopes and dreams for the future, so that you have a clear yardstick to measure your future progress.

One way to do this visioning is to draw a single card from a tarot deck. For example, suppose you inquire about your future self, and you draw the King of Pentacles card. This card is usually associated with material success, as in success in business. It is also associated with keeping your word and being a trusted associate. The card usually depicts the King sitting on a luxurious throne, often with clusters of grapes or a hoard of coins.

Sit with the card for a few minutes, letting its imagery work on you. Keep gazing on the imagery until you can see it with your eyes closed. Now ask yourself a set of questions:

- What is this card telling me that I want for my own future?
- What would I need to let go in order to have the future that I want?
- What factors already exist in my life that will help my vision to become a reality?

Answer these questions in your magickal record. For example, you might write that the card is saying you seek a life of material abundance with great success in business. You might need to let go of a tendency to downplay or neglect your material needs. And you might already have several factors contributing to your success, such as a stable career, a supportive family, or important talents and interests.

Once you have read the card, or allowed the card to read you, get even more specific about your vision. Ask yourself clarifying questions that expand upon the answers you already gave. These clarifying questions might look like the following:

- What kind of lifestyle would I like to have? What would my work habits look like?
- What kind of friends would I keep? Are there specific people I would like to get to know?
- What kinds of material possessions would I own? Where would I live?

Write the answers to these questions in your magickal record, making them as detailed and specific as possible. For example, you might write that you desire to make a living as a freelance artist, working part-time while living in a cabin in the Maine woods.

Don't dismiss your ideas because they seem too far-fetched or impractical. Now is the time for visioning your ideal life.

You also do not need to worry about how your dreams will come true. Your job now is simply to hold a vision there for the cosmos to accept. When you have written down your vision, set it aside for now. Return to it periodically and keep track of any movement toward your goals.

Step 4: Into the Unknown

In the last chapter, you looked at one of the tarot cards for endings and new beginnings, a card like Death, the Tower, Judgement, or the World. It is worth remembering that each and every day, something dies and something else comes to life. Your skin dies and replaces itself entirely every twenty-seven days or so. In fact, your body replaces billions of cells every single day. Even your bones, which seem so solid, are always being broken down and remolded, so that the entire skeleton is replaced every ten years.

You seem to have continuity from day to day, but in reality, everything about yourself changes. And yet, you often wake up in the morning with a feeling that you know what to expect, that you know with a large degree of certainty what will transpire.

Sometimes this expectation of routine becomes self-fulfilling. You can easily fall into the same habits from one day to the next, which produces the feeling of sameness and repetition. These habits greatly simplify life, in that they limit the number of choices you have to make in a given day, but they can also produce blandness and boredom.

To reclaim a sense of the new and unknown waiting for you each day, oppose the customs and habits you have set for yourself. Dedicate yourself to finding new pathways through life. Practice random belief using a random religion generator. Read a new poet or political philosophy. Wear clothes you wouldn't ordinarily wear. Talk to strangers. Park backwards in your driveway. Listen to new music. Read a book from back to front. Cut apart a book and reassemble it. Cut apart your magickal record and reassemble it. Move around the furniture in your house. Try eating new foods, even some that you don't like. Read a random Wikipedia entry. Visit a new town. Sleep outside. Eat dessert first.

In addition to these acts of spontaneity, remind yourself that this is all temporary. Carry the Death card around in your pocket and gaze upon it periodically. Take the time to converse with your departed relatives, and ask them what they would do differently if they could live life all over again. If you have difficulty feeling connected, try cooking some of the foods that they once enjoyed, or try to find a perfume or cologne that was special to them. Play some of the music that your loved one would recognize. Visit their grave if you can, or visit the place where they once lived. Read books about near death experiences and reincarnation. Read books about death and dying.

Part of the chaos tendency is also detachment from the old order and a preparation for the unknown. To that end, make a preparation for new things to come into your life. This means keeping your financial house in order. Make a serious effort to pay off old accounts and close books you are no longer using. If you have any outstanding projects around the house or in your creative or professional life, make sure to finish that work. If you have put off any social contacts, make sure to keep your relationships in good working order. The point here is to live as though you are prepared for death, not that you are literally going to die anytime soon.

When you live in this way, you are prepared for any new thing that might come your way. When your affairs are in order, you can pick up and move to a new city. You can afford to take a little bit of time off for a vacation or creative endeavors. You can take the time to do a longer magickal work. Perhaps you can begin to say the chaos invocation regularly, for thirty, sixty, or ninety days. Perhaps you begin to form magickal associations with people who are on the same path. You can begin to compare notes and share tips with your fellow chaos practitioners.

The point here is that chaos and order go hand in hand. Following the path of chaos does not mean having disorder in every aspect of your life. It is perfectly well and good to control what you can control, to keep the Saturnine/Ketu tendencies toward cold, contracting energy in some areas at least. It is okay to bind some things so that other things can be loosened. When you try to do everything all at once, it leads to a dispersal of energy, which ultimately weakens your concentration and focus. Getting familiar with death and allowing some projects to come to a close will free your hand for the new.

Step 5: Chaos Being

The control society has a tendency to teach the notion of a unitary self—that you should be the same person at all times and in all contexts. Supposedly, to live with integrity means to have no secrets or mysteries, to be the same person at work as at home, in personal and professional life. But this sort of unitary version of the self actually flattens and removes all of the texture from life. As you embark upon the chaos journey, you will find yourself no longer striving for that monolithic vision. You will become more comfortable with your own contradictions and oddities, your hidden aspects and eccentricities.

Your chaos being lives comfortably with the animal aspects of life—with food, drink, and sex—while acknowledging also the artistic and spiritual values and the life of the mind. You need no longer distinguish between "high" and "low" culture, between the things of the soul and the things of the flesh. Nor do you need to seek a synthesis or fusion between competing sets of values. The chaos path works well with amalgamation, with juxtaposition, with disharmony and discord. You can simply acknowledge certain irreconcilable facts about yourself. You need not be the same person tomorrow that you were today. The past no longer holds you.

Take the time now to write down three ways that the chaos tendency has affected you. You might find that new people, things, or ideas have entered your life since you began reading this book. You may be finding that some of your old habits no longer serve you, and you might be more willing to change your basic outlook toward life. Maybe even some things that you once considered nonnegotiable now seem up for grabs. Also, write down some changes that you feel like might be on the cusp of arriving.

Think also about your queer ancestors or chosen family. As you think about their creative works and their lives, what would they want for you now? And think also of the queer people in your life right now. What would queer liberation look like if you were to make it more significant in your life?

Imagine that queer liberation and chaos magick are one and the same process. Spend some time writing in your journal about what you want for your queer self, how you can be more expansive in your definition of your gender, your sexuality, your personality, and your identity.

Magick works through life itself, and life ends too soon. As earthbound creatures, we have to go after the things that we want right away, without the least hesitation. The energy you put into the saying of spells and crafting of sigils will be the same intensity with which you live your everyday life.

Each little action, each thought and feeling, has power and promise in it. The tiniest effort matters and casts its effect into the universe. Everything that we do each day holds magick in it: we just have to approach life with the passionate drive for growth and exploration.

An Ending and a Beginning

In this chapter, you learned to invoke chaos directly through its 108 names. You gazed into the broken mirror and saw branching lines of possibility extending from the past to the present to the future. You saw the many ways in which you are living into your highest potential and entered into the mystery at the heart of existence. You learned to encounter your shadow side and made space for all of the versions of yourself to enter into the light.

You have also learned to reflect on death, endings, and new beginnings as you contemplated what no longer serves you and what you want to invite into your world. You recalled your queer ancestors and chosen family and resolved to live a bolder version of your life. And you resolved to live to the fullest, knowing the fleeting nature of earthly existence.

In the days, weeks, months, and years ahead, you will have many more opportunities to harness the power of chaos and live into your full potential. Go forward boldly, knowing that you are already one with the queer force of change at the heart of all things. The future unfolds according to the dictates of your own imagination.

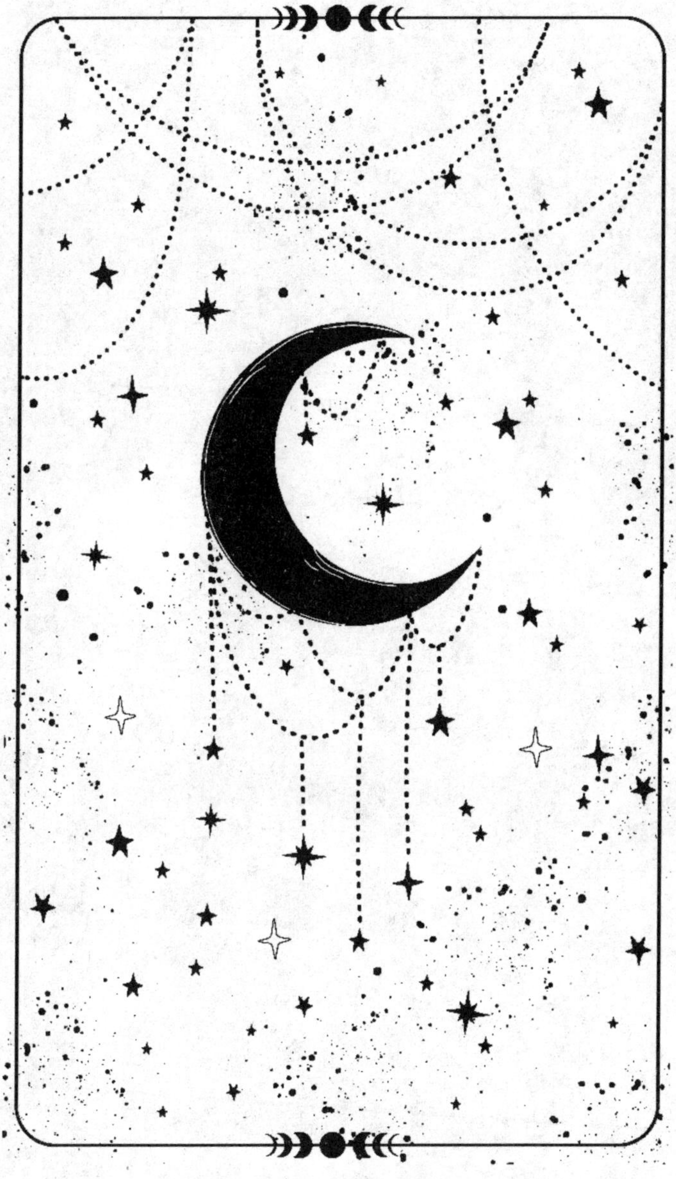

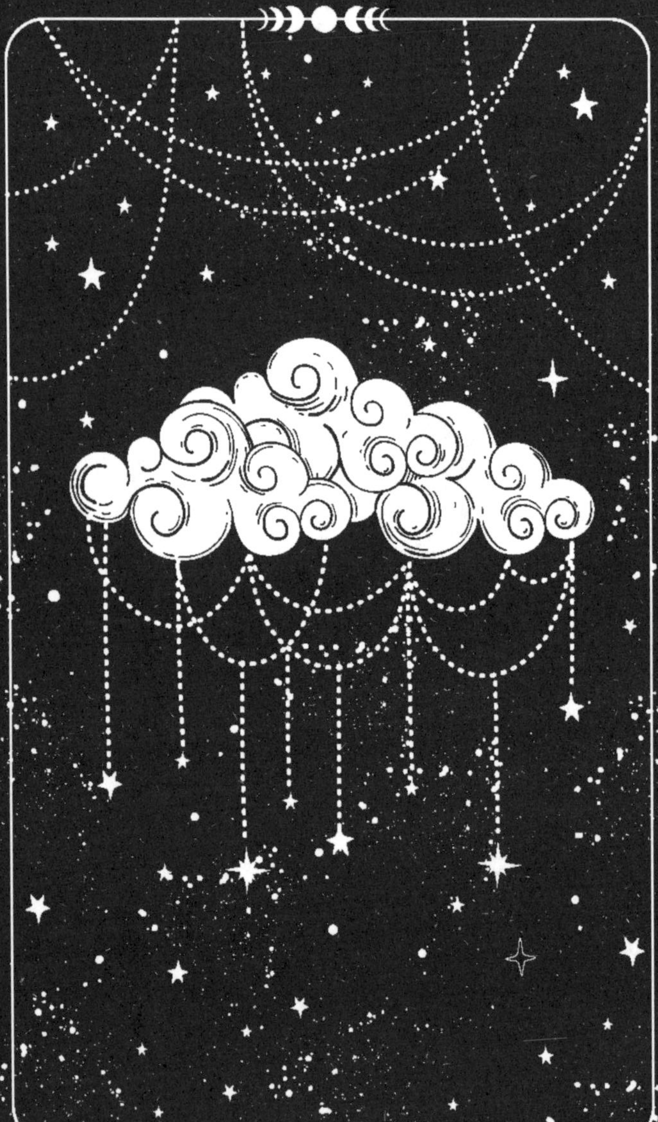

Conclusion

On your journey as a queer person, as a witch, mage, rootworker, herbalist, magician, or mystic, you may have been told outright that you were simply too much or too dramatic, that you were unacceptable or embarrassing, that you were lying or faking it, that you were sinful or unseemly.

Patriarchy, racism, homophobia, and ableism are all about enforcing the dominant order, and anyone who falls on the wrong side of that order will be excluded or castigated. Chaos magicians stand with those who fall on the wrong side of the ledger, with the unruly waters on the other side of the firmament. We cannot be properly controlled or governed. We do not fit. We do not acquiesce.

You have come so far on a long journey of self-discovery and ritual empowerment. At the beginning of this work, you came to see the universe itself as queer and dedicated your magickal record. Then, you learned to enter the chaosphere and get in touch with your true will. You learned to connect with your true desires and crafted a sigil to bring your fantasies into reality. You did a lot of work on embodiment, getting to know and appreciate all parts of your physical form and doing a ritual to banish shame. You found your true will and learned planetary divination and automatic writing for any purpose. You learned scrying, visualization, and telepathy. And finally, you invoked chaos herself as a great goddess and enlisted her help to revivify the tired commonplaceness of life.

As I finish writing this book at the beginning of March, the snow is falling on Western Massachusetts. Tonight will be the Worm Moon, the full moon named for the earthworms who are restarting their activity in anticipation of spring. It is also called the Sap Moon or the Sugar Moon, named for the maple syrup season which is now in full swing. It could snow five to eight inches today, but I know that the seasons are changing. Soon, I will be drinking coffee with my wife on the patio before work. Our lives go through seasons, ups and downs, hard times and easy times, happy times and sad times.

Chaos magick is about control to a certain extent, trying to make things happen, but it is also about relinquishing the need to control, to just enjoy this chaotic universe and be one with it.

It is also about escaping from control, from those societal messages that threaten us as queer people. We practice in solitude, but we also practice with and for each other, in solidarity with all people who are marginalized and excluded.

Take from this book whatever is good and useful. Embrace the dark light of chaos, and circumstances will become more bearable and malleable. No matter how difficult things may seem, take the power you do have and live into your true will.

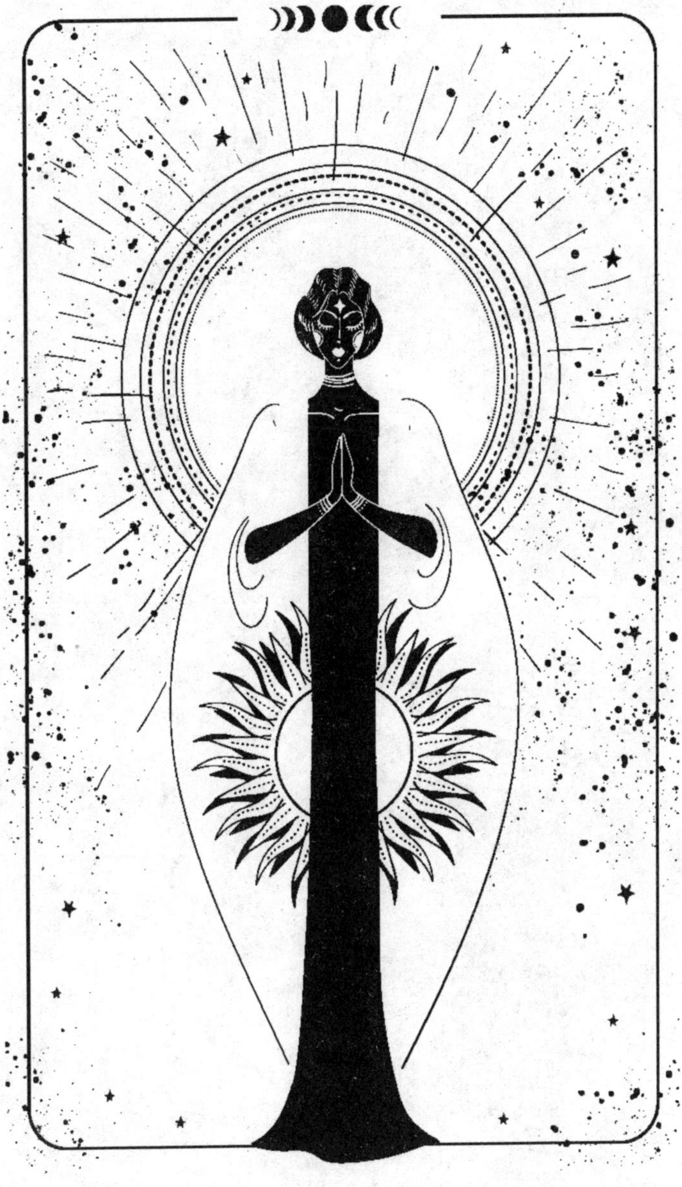

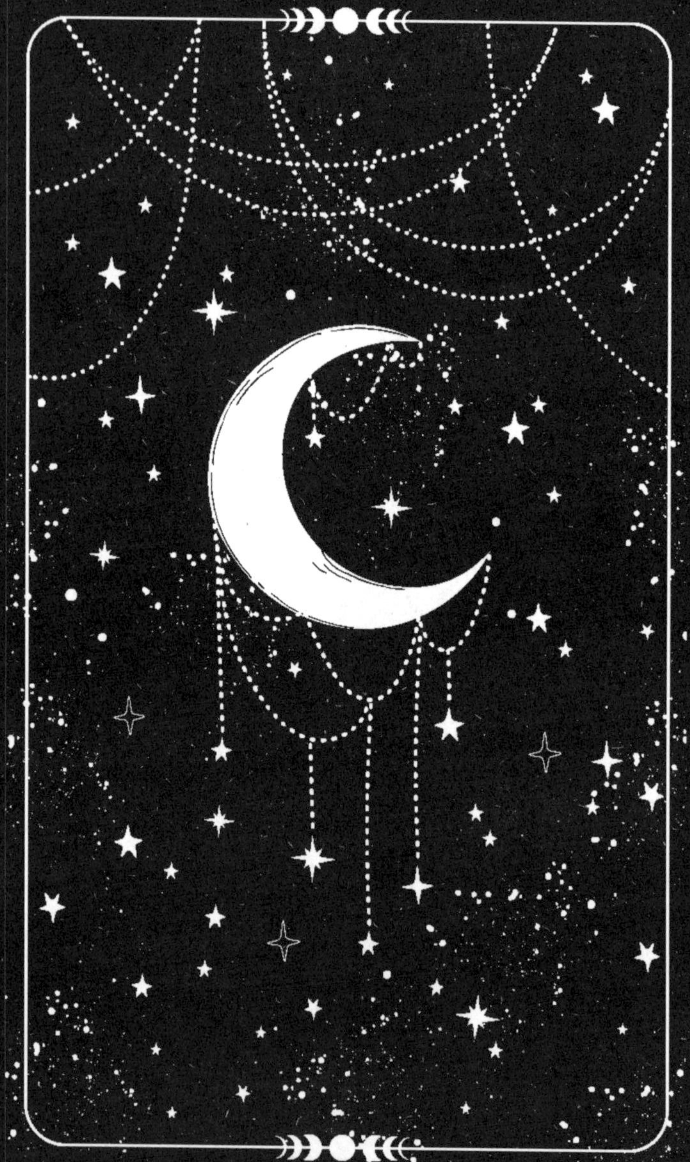

References and Further Reading

Carroll, Peter. *Liber Null and Psychonaut.* York Beach, ME: Weiser, 1987.

Conway, D.J. *A Little Book of Pendulum Magic.* New York: Crossing Press, 2001.

Crowley, Aleister. *The Book of the Law / Liber Al Vel Legis.* Newburyport, MA: Red Wheel/Weiser, 2004.

—. *Gems from the Equinox: Instructions by Aleister Crowley for His Own Magickal Order.* Newburyport, MA: Weiser, 2007.

Dee, Steve. "The Queer Gods of Alchemy." In *Queer Magic: Power Beyond Boundaries.* Ed. Lee Harrington and Tai Fenix Kulystin. Anchorage, AK: Mystic Productions, 2018. 54–63.

Duggan, Colin. "Chaos Magick." In *The Occult World.* Ed. Christopher Partridge. Routledge, London: 2014. 406–411.

Goddard, Neville. *Infinite Potential: The Greatest Works of Neville Goddard.* Ed. Mitch Horowitz. New York: St. Martin's, 2019.

Hedva, Johanna. *How to Tell When We Will Die: On Pain, Disability, and Doom.* New York: Hillman Grad, 2024.

Heineman, Kristin. "Why Are There 7 Days in a Week? Thank the Babylonians." *Astronomy,* January 25, 2024. https://www.astronomy.com/science/

why-are-there-7-days-in-a-week-thank-the-babylonians/

Hine, Phil. *Condensed Chaos: An Introduction to Chaos Magic.* Tempe, AZ: New Falcon, 1995.

Horowitz, Mitch. *The Miracle Club: How Thoughts Become Reality.* Rochester, VT: Inner Traditions, 2018.

—. *Magician of the Beautiful: An Introduction to Neville Goddard.* New York: Gildan Media, 2019.

Kirby, Danielle. "Occultural Bricolage and Popular Culture: Remix and Art in Discordianism, the Church of the Subgenius, and The Temple of Psychick Youth." *Handbook of Hyper-Real Religions.* Leiden: Brill, 2012. 37–57.

Parma, Fio Gede. *The Witch Belongs to the World: A Spell of Becoming.* Woodbury, MN: Llewellyn, 2023.

P-Orridge, Genesis Breyer. *Thee Psychick Bible: Thee Apocryphal Scriptures ov Genesis Breyer P-Orridge and Thee Third Mind ov Thee Temple of Psychick Youth.* Port Townsend, WA: Feral House, 2009.

Prower, Tomás. *Queer Magic: LGBT+ Spirituality and Culture from Around the World.* Woodbury, MN: Llewellyn, 2018.

Sinclair, Vanessa and Carl Abrahamsson. *It's Magic Monday Every Day of the Week.* Vimmerby, Sweden: Trapart Books, 2021.

Snow, Cassandra. *Queering Your Craft: Witchcraft from the Margins.* Newburyport, MA: Red Wheel/Weiser, 2020.

Vitimus, Andrieh. *Hands-On Chaos Magick: Reality Manipulation through the Ovayki Current.* Woodbury, MN: Llewellyn, 2009.

Wachter, Aidan. *Six Ways: Approaches and Entries for Practical Magic.* Ygret Niche Publishing, 2018.

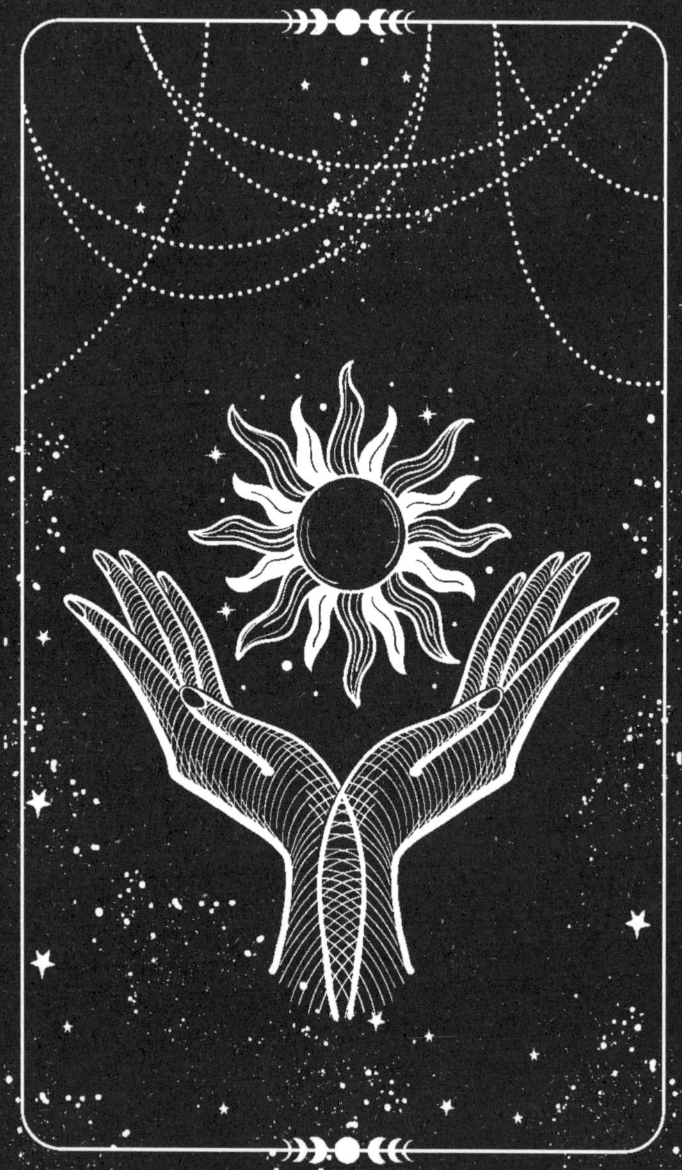

About the Author

Devi Dillard-Wright, Ph.D., is the author of Self-Love: 100+ Quotes, Reflections, and Activities to Help You Uncover and Strengthen Your Self-Love, as well as many other books on mindfulness in daily life. Devi taught philosophy for over fifteen years at the University of South Carolina Aiken and now teaches English as a Second Language in Western Massachusetts. Find her on X/ Twitter @DBDillardWright.

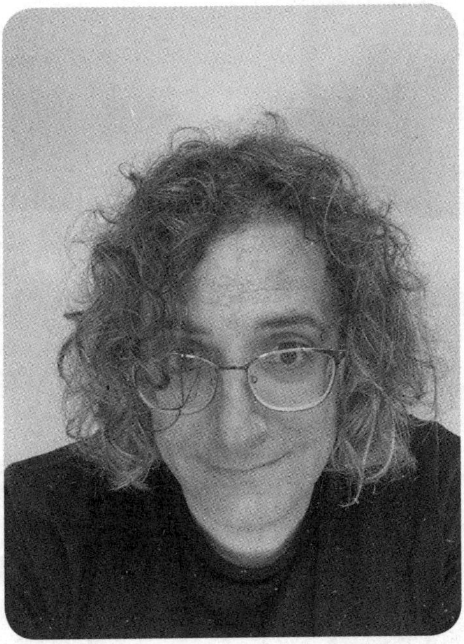

FIND MORE MAGIC AT MICROCOSM.PUB

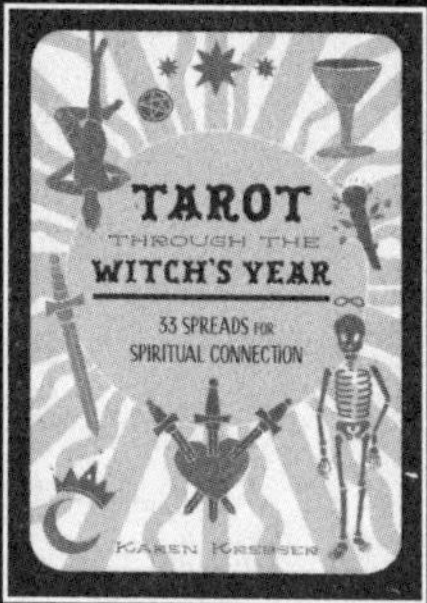

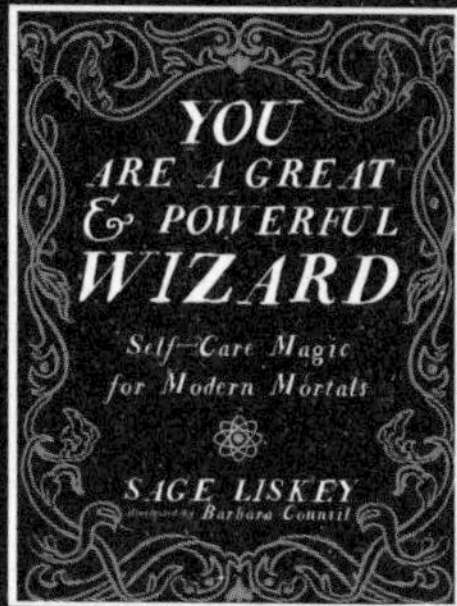

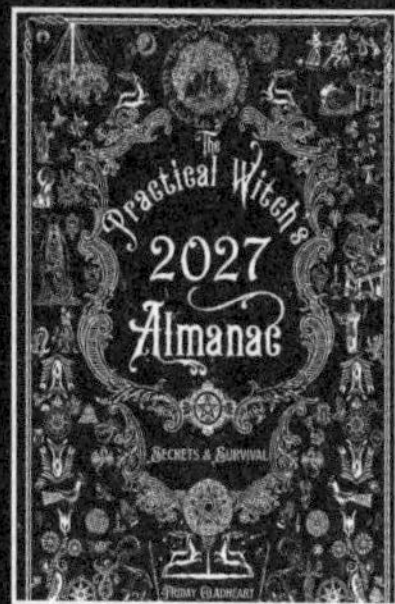

SUBSCRIBE!

For as little as $15/month, you can support a small, independent publisher and get every book that we publish—

delivered to your doorstep!

www.Microcosm.Pub/BFF

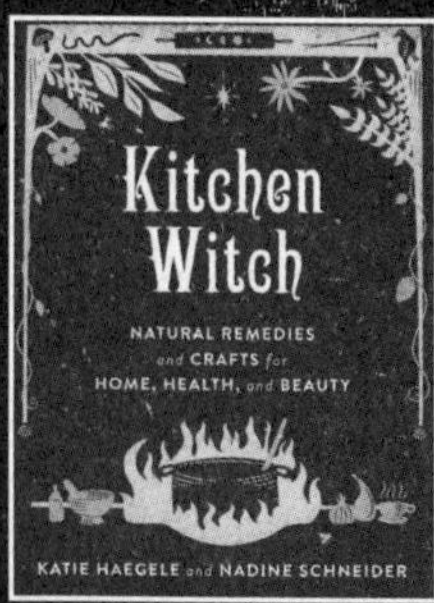